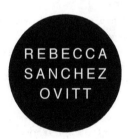

My Journey

of Healing from Cancer

REBECCA
SANCHEZ
OVITT

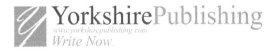

YorkshirePublishing
www.yorkshirepublishing.com
Write Now.

ISBN: 978-1-947491-77-9
My Journey of Healing from Cancer
Copyright © 2006 by Rebecca Sanchez Ovitt

Unless otherwise noted Scripture quotations are taken from the Holy Bible, New International Version ®, Copyright © 1973, 1978, 1984, 1985 by International Bible Society. Used by permission of Zondervan Publishing House. All rights reserved.

Scripture quotations marked "KJV" are taken from the Holy Bible, King James Version, Cambridge, 1769.

Cover and interior design by Lindsay B. Behrens

For permission requests, write to the publisher at the address below.

Yorkshire Publishing
3207 South Norwood Avenue
Tulsa, Oklahoma 74135
www.YorkshirePublishing.com
918.394.2665

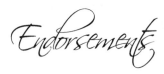
Endorsements

"A must read for all those going through cancer who want to know there is hope! Dr. Ovitt takes you through the very heart of suffering with embraces of love and hope."
Hale Akamine
PhD, Clinical Psychologist

"Cancer is a difficult diagnosis to accept no matter who you are. This book is an inspiration to anyone undergoing the most arduous stage in one's life. With God's love, one can accept the diagnosis and have courage to move on and recover from this devastating disease with strength."
Cheryl P. Sanchez-Kazi, MD, FAAP, FASN
University of Wisconsin School of Medicine and Public Health

"A truly genuine, honest, and touching narrative of a woman's experiences as she fights the greatest battle of her life—ovarian cancer. Dr. Ovitt is testimony that with faith in God, we can survive even the toughest challenges of our lives. Reading the book puts the reader in the same room as the patient."
Remee Bolante
Vice-Principal, Sacred Hearts Academy

"A journey…pain…suffering…fear…strength…joy…tenderness inspira-tion…the author takes you through her journey of cancer and the reader ends up seeing a glimpse of God, experiencing how He holds our hands and carries

us, even in our most vulnerable and painful times of life. There is victory…an inspiration to anyone who is suffering."
Pat Murphy
Counselor

"Dr. Ovitt's message of unconditional love and unending hope will impact the lives of people facing cancer diagnosis and possible terminal illness. This includes their families and friends as well as their health care providers. Trusting God's plan and embracing life with love and compassion, yes, this is the very essence of Ovitt's journey."
Ines Bejarin Finin, RN, MS
Clinical Nurse Specialist, Kapiolani Breast Center
Adjunct Faculty, Hawaii Pacific University, College of Nursing

"This captivating story of Dr. Rebecca Sanchez Ovitt exemplifies God's amazing grace, love and healing. I highly recommend this inspiring book, which will be a great help and encouragement to anyone facing trials and tribulations of any kind. Powerful living words from the Bible will give you strength and hope to live victoriously."
Deanna C. Aoki
Woman's Missionary Union and Family Ministries Leader
Hawaii Pacific Baptist Convention

"Whether one has had cancer or not, the reading of this book will be a personal blessing. The author documents her journey through surgery, the diagnosis of cancer and the terrors of chemotherapy. Through it all she finds God is there every step of the way, encouraging, loving and strengthening her."
Betty Koon Petherbridge
Bible teacher and retired Private Elementary School teacher

"Through her painful ordeal, Dr. Ovitt continues to be the strong person I have known—spiritually and emotionally. Her powerful personal testimony will draw others to the Lord. I am glad to be one of her friends."
Stan Sagert
President Emeritus, Hawaii Baptist Academy
Retired Colonel, USAF

"Ruby Ovitt's touching testimony of God's grace through her ordeal with cancer reflects the woman I have known for 30 years—warm, authentic, not self-pitying but people-oriented and God-honoring. She could have died, but God kept her going to share her story to help reinforce our faith in His goodness."

Ada Lum
Bible Study trainer with International Fellowship of Evangelical Students and Bible Institute of Hawaii

"Dr. Ovitt's personal testimony is a dynamic inspirational story that challenges all believers to continue to follow God in all circumstances. A must read for those involved in pastoral care ministry to families. This book made me realize that life is fragile."

Rev. Robert Whitfield
Donor Relations/International Relations, Dallas Baptist University

"You cannot read this book without being profoundly moved. The reader literally walks with Dr. Ovitt on an intimate journey and discovers that the peripheries of life are no longer of ultimate concern. After reading her book I was struck by one thought: the more aware we are of our human needs the more overwhelmed we are of our need for God."

Dr. Timothy T. Morita
Vice President for Institutional Advancement, Hawaii Baptist Academy
Retired Navy Captain, Chaplain Corps

"This book is a powerful story of Dr. Ovitt's faith in God during her battle with cancer, the most difficult time in her life. This will bring inspiration and encouragement to others. I highly recommend it."

Sharon Butac
Secretary

"God is truly good. My heart cried and rejoiced as Ruby shared her intimate battle with cancer. In her valley, Ruby helped me see the power of God, the love of God, and her faith in God."

Mark Sugimoto
Superintendent of Hanalani Schools

"Ruby Ovitt is God's broken vessel, repaired by Him to do His will. Stay the course, Ruby!"
Henry Whitehead
Architect, Stone Mountain, Georgia

"Dr. Ovitt's faith and trust is as solid as a rock. Saint Peter's was also and we can see how God used him. This is a wonderful testimony."
Christine H. Whitehead
housewife, Stone Mountain, Georgia

Dedication

This book is lovingly dedicated to my Lord, Jesus Christ,

and to my children,

Christopher and Rochelle

Acknowledgments

This book would not have been possible without the love, prayers, support and encouragement of my beloved children, Christopher and Rochelle; other family members on the East and West Coast, USA, and in the Philippines, especially my sister, Lourdes, brothers, Joe and Junior, sister-in-law, Sofing, mother-in-law, Evelyn, and ex-husband, Dwight.

A very special "mahalo" thank you to the teachers, staff, students, and parents of Hawaii Baptist Academy for the hundreds of letters, cards, drawings, DVDs, CDs, and other expressions of their love and kindness and their prayers throughout my ordeal; to the prayerful members of my church, University Avenue Baptist Church; to friends at the Bible Institute of Hawaii; to the loving members of my Support Group; to friends and colleagues at the Hawaii Association of Independent Schools and Hawaii Council of Private Schools; to friends at the East-West Center Alumni Association; to my compassionate Bible Study and Prayer Group; and other loving friends in the Lord.

A special thank you, too, to my doctors, nurses, health aides and other care givers at Kaiser Hospital in Moanalua who helped me get better and encouraged me in my journey of recovery.

A heartfelt thank you to Mrs. Betty Petherbridge, who edited my drafts and continually encouraged and prayed for me in the completion of this project.

And to all those who have cancer and are journeying with the Lord toward their healing, I send my love and prayers. May your faith remain strong in the Lord!

Introduction

On February 6, 2005, one day after my surgery to remove a large tumor in my left ovary, I was informed by the doctor who operated on me that I had ovarian cancer, the aggressive type! The news was a big surprise to me because I did not have any symptoms of my illness. I even did my regular walking exercise and attended to my responsibilities at school the day before my son took me to the emergency. I thought I was healthy.

One month after my surgery, I underwent chemotherapy treatments every four weeks for four hours each treatment and persevered all the side effects of the cancer drug. I felt all was well until an infection of my gallbladder was diagnosed. I underwent surgery again to remove it on June 17, 2005. The chemotherapy treatments were postponed and resumed on August 9, 2005 and the final treatment was completed in September 2005. The two surgeries weakened my body but not my spirit.

My experiences about my two surgeries, the finding out that I had ovarian cancer, my chemotherapy treatments, and my struggles to overcome physical, mental and emotional pain provided me a much deeper understanding of my relationship with my Lord and Savior, Jesus Christ. I began to write my thoughts and feelings about my walk with Him during my ordeal and the result is this book.

I want to share with you how when I reached out to God in the midst of my pain He gave me mercy; how I felt His presence when He touched me and calmed my spirit when I learned that I had cancer; how He gave me strength and comfort when I was very weak physically and emotionally; how I fully embraced His promise that I have an everlasting life with Him; how I should take care of my body because it is His temple and how blessed I am for this; how I learned that there are times when things happen beyond my control but only He can give me hope; how when I failed to focus on Him, I began to lose my perspective of what is truly essential, my relationship with Him; how I was blessed by the prayers, love, support, encouragement, compassion and kindness of so many people because they wanted to express God's love and I am connected to them through His love; how praying continually for others brought peace to my aching heart; how I praised Him for giving me opportunities to share about His love even in my pain; how I thanked Him in my battle of cancer; and how being His child and being still gave me joy and courage to face the future.

I included some Bible verses that helped me and hopefully these verses will help you, too. I also discussed how one could become a Christian. Perhaps someone wants to become one. I pray that this will happen.

I added some cinquain poetry that describes some of my feelings on some topics and ended this book with a poem that overall reflects my thoughts and feelings about my physical and emotional condition and my walk with God.

My journey toward healing drew me even closer to God. He is truly number one in my life and nothing can separate me from Him. My faith blossomed and I feel so blessed. How wonderful to be His child!

I hope that by reading this book, you will be further strengthened in your faith as you walk with God during a painful experience in your life. As you continue to love Him and keep on holding His Hands, you will have joy in the midst of your pain. Our Lord is faithful and you will be comforted by His presence during your journey toward healing. God bless you, my dear brothers and sisters in Christ.

Honolulu, Hawaii
November 15, 2005

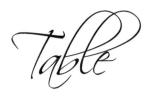

# of Contents

Endorsements 3

Dedication 7

Acknowledgements 9

Introduction 11

1.   Mercy Versus Self-Pity 16

2.   The Journey Begins 20

3.   A Small Triumphant Walk 24

4.   Blessed Assurance 28

5.   God's Temple 32

6.   Joyful Hope 40

7.   Fear and Serenity 44

8.   Connected Through God's Love 48

9. A Peaceful Heart 56

10. Song of Praise 62

11. A Thankful Heart 72

12. Being Still 76

13. Some Bible Verses That Were Helpful to Me 85

14. How Does One Become a Christian? 90

15. Cinquain Poetry 93

16. Epilogue: A Cancer Patient's Prayer 95

Bibliography 101

"Praise be the Lord,

for he has heard

my cry

for mercy."

(Psalm 28:6)

Mercy
Versus Self-Pity

It was 9:00 o'clock in the evening. I was in the emergency room of Kaiser Hospital in Moanalua trying not to groan unlike the man and woman on the left and right side of my bed. The pain on the left side of my abdomen continued to intensify. It started as a dull pain at 3:00 o'clock that afternoon and it continued escalating. I tried to massage the spot gently but it did not help. The pain kept coming like the endless waves trying to reach the shore.

I closed my eyes and mouth tightly to stop thinking of the pain. Suddenly I was startled by the man shouting at the nurses. "Leave me alone! Don't touch me! You only make it worse!" And he kept shouting over and over. I found myself praying. "Lord, please help him. Please help all of us here in this room."

In that small and busy emergency room where several doctors, nurses and others were attending to patients, I felt so alone. It seemed like I was in a small boat drifting in the middle of the ocean with no island in sight. No one had come to attend to me and I was in severe pain. Perhaps if I would shout like the man next to me, someone would attend to me immediately. It seemed like I had been waiting for someone to attend to me forever. I cried silently. I felt so sorry for myself. Then I caught myself. I was experiencing self-pity! "Oh Lord, I do not want self-pity. This is not good for me to dwell on. I need Your mercy instead of self-pity. Lord, please have mercy on me. Please let me feel Your presence and help me to bear this intense pain," I prayed silently. Soon afterwards, I felt calm and slowly began to accept my emotional and physical condition. I tried to focus on God's mercy so I could bear the pain.

About an hour later, I felt a warm hand touch my hand and a gentle voice said, "Mrs. Ovitt, we will now take you to the cat scan room. We will try to find out what is causing your pain."

As I was being wheeled to that room, I closed my eyes. I embraced God's mercy and let go of self-pity. Deep inside, I began to feel peaceful and strong.

"Even though I walk

through the valley of the shadow of death,

I will fear no evil,

for you are with me;

your rod and your staff,

they comfort me."

(Psalm 23:4)

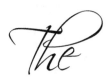

Journey Begins

My surgery was scheduled for 2:00 o'clock in the afternoon on February 5, 2005. At around 1:30, a male nurse came to get me from my room. He rolled the gurney toward the fifth floor where the operating room was located. My two children, my brother and his wife and a dear friend followed us. As the nurse and I were about to enter the waiting area of the operating room, I looked back at them standing a few feet away. I saw their tears and sad faces. I tried to smile and waved at them.

Once inside, my two doctors, Dr. Hirabayashi and Dr. de Bussey, the consultant, Dr. Terada, and the anesthesiologist came by my bedside one at a time and assured me that they will do their best to help me. When they left, I closed my eyes and prayed fervently, "Oh my Jesus, only You know the outcome of this surgery. Please be with the doctors and nurses. Please be with my loved ones. Please calm their spirits and mine, too. Lord, if You decide to take me now, I am ready. Thank You for the many years You have given me. Thank You for my life. My life is in Your hands." I had peace.

The next thing I remembered in my semi-conscious state was I was back in my room and was asking the nurse to let me use the bathroom. I also remembered my son holding my hands saying repeatedly, "We love you, Mommy. We love you, Mommy." I felt very good to hear his affirmations of love.

The following morning, I woke up with severe pain around my stomach area. I asked for a pain killer. The nurse told me to press the small button hanging next to my bed and a small dose of morphine would flow through my veins and would give me relief. "What good news!" I told her. She smiled.

At noon time, Dr. Kimie Hirabayashi came in to see me. She had the sweetest smile and a pleasant personality. After checking my record and status, she looked at me and said calmly, "Mrs. Ovitt, I want you to know about your surgery. You have ovarian cancer, the aggressive type." She stopped talking and we looked at each other silently. Suddenly, a soft and very light warm feeling enveloped my whole being. I felt calm. Then I felt as if someone was gently holding my hands and I heard a soft whisper saying, "I am here. It is alright. I will not leave you." I felt God's presence! While I was still in awe of this wonderful experience and still silent, my doctor proceeded to tell me the extent of my physical illness. She told me that her team found a big cancerous tumor about 5 inches in diameter in my left ovary and the cancer had spread to the left fallopian tube and uterus also. She also told me that the tumor ruptured during surgery and I had a full hysterectomy. There was also the good news that the right ovary, fallopian tube and uterus were free of cancer cells. I was in Stage II–C. She added that I would have to undergo chemotherapy and another doctor would be handling this treatment. Before she left, I thanked her and the other doctors for the job they did to help me. I also told her how much I appreciated her warmth and gentleness.

When I continued to rest in bed, my heart was bursting with joy because I experienced something wonderful, God's presence during one of my life's painful event! I experienced His love and assurance when He gently touched my hands and whispered His comforting words. I received the news about having cancer with calmness and I accepted it. I had peace and was not afraid. Also for the first time in my life, I found out that I was ready to be with Him had He decided to take me during surgery. Furthermore, He had extended my life! Hallelujah for His love for me! I would never trade this wonderful and blessed experience for anything else in this world.

With a joyful heart, I said this prayer. "Lord, thank You for loving me. Thank You for the awesome experience You let me have with You! Thank You for continuing to give me Life! Lord, please be with me as I begin my walk through this valley to combat cancer. This road is unknown to me but You know it fully well. If I falter, hesitate, cry, feel anxious, sad, afraid, angry, depressed, discouraged or whatever, please keep holding me. Lord, You are the Great Physician and I know that You will heal me completely. I put my complete trust in You. Please help and guide the doctors and nurses who will be helping me and also my family. Please help me to have a positive attitude and also to have patience and determination to help myself. Help me to have knowledge and understanding about my physical condition so that I can be an active participant in my healing. If Satan hurls negative thoughts at me, please help me to vanquish them with Your power. You already have victory over him. Help me to discern how this experience can further Your overall plan for my life so that I can bring honor to You. Lord, may I continue to learn and grow in knowing You more as I walk with You through the recovery of my cancer. My strength, comfort and hope are in You, Lord!" After praying, a sweet feeling of assurance filled my heart. That night I slept like a baby.

"But they that wait upon the Lord

shall renew their strength;

they shall mount up with wings as eagles;

they shall run, and not be weary;

and they shall walk,

and not faint."

(Isaiah 40:31, KJV)

Small Triumphant Walk

I was having breakfast when the nurse came in and told me that I had to begin my walking exercise. Immediately after breakfast, she came to help me. It was very painful for me to get out of bed and I found it equally hard to stand steadily. The thought of my walking made me dread the experience; however, I was determined to get better so I took this walking exercise as a challenge. Once standing, she instructed me on how to roll the IV stand and how to hold on to her so I would not fall down.

As we got out of my room, my two children appeared at the end of the hallway. "Mom!" they shouted and they ran toward me to give me a hug. "What are you doing out here?" my son, Chris, asked. The nurse explained to them that walking would be very good for my circulation, strengthen and heal my stomach area and release gas. "Let me help her," Chris said and he took the nurse's place. As I took one small step, my son praised me. "That's good! That's good! One more step, Mommy. Give me one more step." And I did one small step at a time. After about ten minutes, I felt exhausted. I asked my son to take me back to my room. He gently helped me to turn around and upon reaching the door he happily announced, "Wow, that was the shortest triumphant walk you did Mommy. I am very proud of you." I gave him a pat on his shoulder.

My daughter, Chelley, lovingly helped me get back in bed. She put my leg massagers back on and covered me with two blankets because I felt cold. She started to give me a shoulder massage. She was equally pleased at my accomplishments. "Next time I will bring your running shoes and we will go running around here," she added. We both laughed.

My children stayed with me the whole day. They decided to limit the time of visitation of friends after they saw how tired I was and the pain I was experiencing. In between watching TV and going out to buy their food, they phoned friends and shared the news about me. They also returned calls of people who had called earlier. I was impressed at how they were handling our family crisis with calmness and maturity.

They decided to leave after I had my dinner. As they hugged and kissed me goodbye, they affirmed their love for me. Chelley said, "We love you, Mommy. God is watching over you. Focus on getting stronger each day. Eat, rest and exercise. Remember, we are in this together. We are not a family without you."

As they waved goodbye, the memories of that time when they were four and six years old flashed back instantly. There were many 'goodbyes' then because they lived with me for three days and the other three days with their father and alternated Saturdays with their father and me. How I hated those 'goodbyes' and how I longed for their coming back to my home. Every night I used to say a prayer to God similar to this one. "Lord, I beg of You not to let me get sick nor die because my children need me. I want to raise them and help them finish their schooling. They are the reason why I try to be physically and emotionally healthy. Please give me strength and wisdom every day. Please comfort and help us as we go through our pain together." As I look back now, I know that my loving Father heard and answered my prayers. With His abundant love and faithfulness, we walked through the divorce experience triumphantly.

And now, we are facing another family crisis. I know, just like in the past, that He will carry us through again triumphantly. It already began with the small triumphant walk I did that morning.

"For God so loved the world,

that he gave his only begotten Son,

that whosoever

believeth in him

should not perish, but have

everlasting life."

(John 3:16, KJV)

Blessed

Assurance

My illness came so suddenly I did not have time to prepare for it. I was in a meeting at school with my teachers at 3:00 o'clock when I felt a dull pain on the left side of my abdomen. I thought it was due to my eating salsa and chips. The pain continued to escalate, and by 9:00 o'clock that evening my son rushed me to the emergency room at Kaiser Hospital in Moanalua. After a series of cat scans, x-rays, consultation among doctors and talking with my son and me, I underwent surgery. The verdict: ovarian cancer, Stage II-C.

While lying in bed after surgery, my thoughts focused on LIFE, its brevity, beauty and fragileness. For the first time in my life I came face to face with my mortality. I remembered what my mother-in-law used to say, "Life is too short; make the most out of it."

Through the years, I have always tried to make each day count. I always tried to execute my daily, monthly and yearly plans to the best of my ability. I even have a list of future plans such as my plans for my children in their pursuit of higher education, my visits to my daughter in Los Angeles, taking a vacation with my son to Europe, helping my school in its second accreditation process, holding my Support Group classes for the broken-hearted, etc. But all these plans are now in mid-air! My present physical condition did not guarantee that I will be able to accomplish these wonderful plans. My future is unknown!

I do not know how many more days, months or years I will live on this planet. Only God knows; no one else.

Facing the reality of my death, I seriously asked myself these questions. "Am I ready to die?"; "Have I walked with God in my life's journey?"; and "Will I be with Him when my final day comes?"

My conversation with my son came to mind. I shared with him that before my surgery I told God that if it was His will to take me then, that I was still very thankful that I had many years spent with my family and others. I was fulfilled as a woman and as a parent. I further told him that I had no regrets because I had lived a full life. He quickly responded. "You have led a good life but not a full life. You have not yet seen Chelley and me get married. You have not held, played and kissed your future grandchildren. When you have done all these, then you can say that you had a full life but not until then. Try to get better, Mom, because I want to see you with your grandchildren."

His remarks made me feel good. I felt happy that I was included in his future dreams. I admitted to him that I wanted very much to see his future wife and children and also his sister's future family. I also told him that only God can determine our respective futures.

In looking back at my life, I was thankful that I came to know Jesus as my personal Lord and Savior at age fifteen. That was one of my difficult years. I wanted good friends and to do well at school. I was trying so hard to "fit in" with my friends who did not feel bad when they made others feel inadequate and unhappy. When I prayed to God, He assured me that it was okay to be alone because I had to be true to myself first. It was then I realized God loved me even when I was trying to find out who I was in Him and in other relationships. He led me to new friends who cared and cheered for me when I had small successes. He helped me become determined to do my best in my studies and to pursue higher education in the United States. As a foreign student at the University of Hawaii, Columbia University and Stanford University, He helped me to understand cross-cultural problems and rise above them. He helped me overcome temptations and held me close to Him when I was lonely. He became my best friend.

As an administrator, He showed me how to become a servant-leader. He taught me the importance of being forthright, compassionate and fair toward others, especially to the children. He gave me insight and wisdom in making decisions that affected the whole school. He peeled off my pride that was keeping me from realizing my full potential. He strengthened my confidence in carrying out my multi-faceted duties and challenging responsibilities.

As someone who has undergone divorce, He held me close to His heart during this darkest and toughest time of my life. He wiped my tears when I cried for help and comforted my aching soul. He helped me to face the feelings of guilt, anger and depression. He gave me hope for a brighter tomorrow. He forgave my sins and healed my broken heart, which in turn helped me to forgive my ex-spouse. He led me to my new beginning with confidence.

As a parent, my most precious role, He taught me how to love my children unconditionally. He helped me to look at them through His eyes. He showed me how I could help build their self-esteem because they were equally hurt by the divorce. Whenever I failed, which happened many times, He encouraged me to keep on learning from my mistakes and accepting and forgiving myself. He continued to help me see my children's unique qualities and how I could support and nurture them to maximize their talents and abilities. He gave me wisdom as I tried to bravely and prayerfully cope with their on-going developmental stages, especially during their teenage years. He made me realize that my children and I are His children and He will never leave us because He is our Father.

I can sincerely say that from the time I became a Christian to the present, I have tried to follow my Lord's footsteps. I have experienced the warmth of His presence because He was my constant companion. I have fully embraced His promise that I will have an everlasting life with Him when I accepted Him into my heart. Although I am not perfect and am still growing as His child, I know without a doubt that I will be in His loving arms when I leave this world. And if my future plans and my son's dreams will not become a reality, I believe that I have led a full life because it is a life spent with Him. Having walked with Him this far, I find my Life's journey meaningful and beautiful. I am forever grateful to Him for the many years I have lived to enjoy my family, friends and others.

When I went to visit and bade goodbye to my 87 year old father before he passed away, I remember vividly what he said to me. "I will see you later in heaven. I will see you there with Jesus." We cried, hugged and kissed. I felt his peace. The blessed assurance that he had then is mine, too.

"Don't you know

that you yourselves are God's temple

and that

God's Spirit lives in you?"

(1 Corinthians 3:16)

God's

Temple

It was 1:00 o'clock in the afternoon of February 10, 2005, when I checked in for my appointment with Dr. Kimie Hirabasyashi, the doctor who operated on me. My brother, sister-in-law and I were eager to find out what she would say about my progress since I had my surgery five days earlier. She greeted me with a sweet smile and once seated she told me that Dr. Clayton Chan would be handling my chemotherapy treatment and I would have to see her one more time once treatment was completed. When she checked my incision and suture, she happily said, "It is healing beautifully. Let me take out the staples now." As she removed the staples, I closed my eyes, counted with my fingers the staples being removed and spoke quietly as she took out one staple at a time, "Thank You Jesus for loving me." She removed 37 staples from my eight-inch incision therefore, thirty-seven 'thank yous' to Jesus. When we left the hospital, my heart was filled with thankfulness for the beautiful healing of my wound.

After being discharged, my brother and his wife offered that I stay with them for a few days at their new home in Kapolei, so that they could give me all the help I needed to regain my health. My children and I were very appreciative of their kind gesture. The peaceful neighborhood, their manicured yard with flowering plants and shrubs and spacious and lush vegetable garden were welcome sights to me. The fresh air invigorated me.

On my first night at their home I sat in my room in pain. My mind went over some events that happened quickly. It started one afternoon when I felt a dull pain on the left side of my abdomen. Two days later, I underwent surgery to remove a big tumor in my left ovary which ruptured and was told I had ovarian cancer, the aggressive type. Then the check up this morning and now the beginning of my recuperation process before chemotherapy treatment would begin in the next few days.

As I recalled these events, warm tears rolled down my cheeks. I cried silently. I remained quiet and savored the quietness around me. I was not fearful or angry at God at what had happened to me. I was crying because my heart was overflowing with thankfulness to God that I came out of surgery alive. I recalled how God held my hands when my doctor told me after surgery I had cancer. I remained quiet and still during that time and told God that I surrendered myself to Him. I knew He was in control of everything. And now in this quiet room, I knew too that the Holy Spirit, who dwells in me, is holding me and giving me the assurance that He will be with me. My body is His temple. I prayed silently, "Lord, thank You that I am Your temple. My body belongs to You. Help me to take care of this temple the best I can in spite of my illness." My prayer brought quietness in my heart. I felt His presence.

For the next few days my mind was focused on what it meant for me to be God's temple. I understand that to be one, my thoughts, feelings and behavior have to be all integrated and aligned with God. What I think, feel and do have to be under God's leading. What my mind thinks will affect my feeling; my feeling will affect my behavior; and my behavior will affect how I will treat my body and how it will respond. They are all interconnected, therefore, any negative thought, feeling, or behavior will be a stumbling block to my healing. I have to be constantly in prayer because it is only through the power of the Holy Spirit working in me that I will be able to align my thoughts, feelings and behavior with Him. My strong faith will give serenity to my soul and the Holy Spirit will empower me to face the future, especially my present circumstance, with peace, confidence, and assurance.

With a thankful heart I offered a prayer, "Lord, thank You for this wonderful assurance that my life is in Your Hands! Thank You that I am special to You because there is no one just like me. You designed my body when I was conceived in my mother's womb. Help me to continue to love, appreciate, take care of, and respect this wonderful body. Help me also to nurture this beautiful mind You have given me. Help me to think of beautiful thoughts about You and others in my present situation. Help me to continue to have good feelings about myself and others. Help me to continually discern what positive actions I have to take during my recuperation. Please help me to overcome any negative thoughts and feelings that may creep into my heart and mind. I beg for Your mercy and grace and I put my complete trust in You for restoring my body. Thank You for living in me. I feel fully blessed."

Deep down in my heart I knew that when I became a Christian, I tried with all my heart and mind to follow God's footsteps, because I wanted to please Him. The fact that I am His temple made me even more aware of my sins, shortcomings and failures. I have asked for His forgiveness of my sins many times. I sought His advice whenever I faced temptation and repented with all my heart when I succumbed to it and rejoiced with gladness when I overcame it. I learned that there is victory in His power! I realized that subjecting my thoughts, feelings and behavior with Him every day was very difficult however, it became possible only when I continually focused my gaze on Him and asked for His strength. Many times when I felt downhearted, because of the negative circumstances I was in and the problems I was facing, I would hear Him say, "I am here, trust me." It was during those times that my heart would swell with confidence and my mind would be filled with wonderful ideas of how I would be able to overcome the negative situations and problems. Through the years, with a grateful heart, I continue to slowly learn how to follow Him. I want to be more loving, giving, trusting and forgiving. I want to have a pure heart. And now that I am facing my battle to beat cancer, I want my whole being to be even more in tune with His heart, as I journey on toward my healing.

The following days, I showed my determination to be an active participant in my own healing. Although I was in pain, I tried to walk even a few steps everyday. I used the walker wherever I went, even to the bathroom, because it was painful and uncomfortable to sit down and stand up. My biggest challenge was getting in and out of bed without help and also lying flat on my back all night, because it was impossible to turn onto either side. When I woke up at night due to pain, in spite of taking some pain medication, I would say a prayer. "Lord, please help me to persevere. Please give me strength and patience." Since I lay awake each night until around one or two in the morning, I decided to study the whole Bible. I used the Bible given to me by a dear friend, *Everyday with Jesus Bible,* 2004 by Holman Bible Publishers, a combination of the Old and New Testament daily Bible study. This helped me tremendously because my mind was focused on God's words rather than on my bodily pain. It gave me peace and assurance that I would get better each day.

I thoroughly enjoyed my stay at Kapolei. My brother and sister-in-law were very sympathetic and attentive to my needs. They prayed and gave me encouraging words everyday. My sister-in-law prepared delicious dishes using fresh vegetables from their garden mixed with meat or fish and served nutritious snacks. She helped me by putting the dressing on my incision. My brother saw to it that I took my naps, did my walking and breathing exercises and gave me shoulder and back massages at night. One of our joys was during mealtime. We shared openly about our past struggles and successes as individuals and parents. The highlight was always my brother's interesting adventures as a young boy during World War II in the Philippines.

When my son came to visit, my brother proudly announced, "Chris, your mom gained two pounds and she is walking a little bit faster now." My son was delighted. "That is good news, Mom! I am sure it's all about Auntie's cooking," he replied as he glanced at my sister-in-law with a big smile. Surely my brother and sister-in-law's kindness, love, and support will forever remain in my heart.

When I returned home, I was very surprised when I saw some changes in the apartment that my children made to make it user-friendly especially for me. They fixed and decorated nicely my son's bedroom, located on the fourth floor, to be my bedroom so that I would not have to climb fifteen steps to go to my former bedroom located on the fifth floor. They also fixed and decorated nicely the bathroom next to it so that it would be more accessible for me, especially at night. They bought a firm queen size bed and put on matching bed sheets and pillows with my favorite colors. They brought down some of my clothes that they thought were appropriate for me during my recuperation and arranged them neatly in the drawers and closet. They put the large TV, VCR, DVD players and I-Pod on top of the big dresser along with several Christian CDs, funny movies and videos. They bought a comfortable chair to match the small table and put on it my Bible, selected books, pens, pencils, papers, stamps, blank cards and address books. They pinned some family pictures and students' drawings on the bulletin board. They moved the location of the microwave and broiler-toaster in the kitchen, re-arranged the entertainment center, and removed some items in the hallway in order to have more space. They did all of these to support my healing. I was deeply moved as I thanked them for their love, hard work, support and encouragement.

When my daughter bade me goodbye to return to Los Angeles, she embraced and kissed me and said, "I am glad that you are happy, Mom. We will do all we can to make you happy so you will get stronger each day. Chris and

I want you to get well because we love you very much. We are always here for you. I will look into buying you a wig and will keep you informed. Do not forget to drink lots of water and eat fresh fruits and vegetables." I gave her a big hug. "Both of you are my angels on earth. What more can I ask? I feel so blessed as your mother," I replied. When she left, my heart was full of love.

After my first chemotherapy treatment, I realized how much bodily pain there was. Oh, the overall feelings of fatigue and muscle pain and other side effects were something to remember. The over-all side effects of this cancer drug on my body made me wonder how people who also have chemotherapy treatment help themselves. I found myself praying for these unknown people, including myself. I asked for God's loving hands to comfort us and help us accept our pain graciously.

As my chemotherapy treatment progressed, I continued to pray. I prayed that I would be able to accept the pain with a thankful heart; that I would have the desire to eat even though the food was tasteless; that I would not become addicted to my pain medication and use it only as needed; that I would be able to think positively whenever I was feeling lonely, sorry for myself and overly anxious. On the days that I had these feelings, I would say what I was thankful for. "Lord, thank You for all the people who are praying for me." "Thank You for the visit of my dear friend." "Thank You for the letters and drawings of the students." "Thank You for the food sent to us." "Thank You for the Worship Network on TV." "Thank You for my sister's phone call." etc. I would keep on giving "thanks" until I felt composed and still. These "thankful prayers" were a powerful antidote for my loneliness and anxiety. I deliberately refused to entertain negative thoughts, because they dampen my spirit and over-all bodily function. As God's temple, I know He wants me to be positive and call on Him all the time.

I tried to be proactive about my needs. I called the pharmacist and asked about the side effects of some medicines that were prescribed for me. If I felt that the side effects would be too much for my body, I would ask for an alternative medicine. I called my doctor or consulted the booklet, *Chemotherapy and You,* and other literature to further understand the side effects of the cancer drug. I checked the internet for more information about ovarian cancer. I read literature that included success stories of people who had overcome ovarian cancer and other kinds of cancer. I cooked foods that were good for me, with the help of my son, and avoided those that would not benefit my healing. I called some people that I knew had cancer and asked how they were handling themselves. I read inspirational materials and books and watched TV shows and videos that made me feel light and happy. I listened to Christian music all the time. I wrote to friends and family and answered some letters. I called and returned phone calls and sent e-mails. I made a flexible schedule for me so that I had some specific activities to accomplish daily, especially my exercise, meditation and Bible study. If for some reason I was not able to accomplish all that was on my list I accepted it without resentment. I tried to be gentle and understanding of my body's needs.

One day my spirit was troubled because of information that I read from literature given by a friend who came to visit me. It contained more information about ovarian cancer. It showed the statistics about the five-year survival rate of women with ovarian cancer in different stages. These are: Stage I, 80–90 percent; Stage II, 65–70 percent; Stage III, 30–60 percent; and Stage IV, 20 percent. It stated that the five-year survival rate was used to provide a standard way of discussing prognosis. It further stated that the figures were approximate, because it varies with the health and age of the patients. Furthermore, the disease can reoccur after the completion of cancer treatment.

What I read affected my positive attitude. The statistics kept coming to my mind! I could not erase it. I felt gloomy. I hardly ate or slept. My heart was gripped with fear and doubt. I felt like I was doomed to die within five years. I prayed day and night for God to deliver me from my depressive outlook. I focused on the many miracles that He had done. He healed so many people, the blind, the lame, the sick and even gave life to someone who died. He had great compassion for those who were sick and He healed them. (Matthew 14:14; Mark 1:34; 3:10) I prayed to God to also show His compassion toward me.

I recalled the story of King Hezekiah in the Old Testament who was a faithful and devoted follower of the Lord. He did mighty works throughout his kingdom and one of these was helping his people to worship God again instead of their idols. He spent his time pleasing the Lord; however, he became gravely ill, and the prophet Isaiah told him that he would die. He wept bitterly and prayed to God. He reminded Him how much he loved and served Him. God heard his prayers, healed him and extended his life for several years. (2Kings 20:1–6) I prayed that He would do the same for me as he had done for King Hezekiah.

The answer to my dilemma came when a friend called to inform me that a mutual friend had died suddenly. We were surprised and saddened, but secure in our thoughts that our friend was already with Jesus in heaven because he had Christ in his heart. We admired his Christian lifestyle. We prayed for his wonderful family.

My talk with my friend opened my eyes that those statistics I was focusing on, that caused me stress and anxiety, were man made and not from God. Man's work, let alone these statistics, is not perfect. God's design for my life is perfect. God can take my life at any time, in whatever stage I am in my illness or whether I have cancer or not. I do not need to be sick from cancer to die. I may die at any time, according to His loving will. He may also extend my life according to His purpose.

This realization lifted my spirit! I knew that I could endure my illness but not a troubled spirit, because it halts my progress toward wholeness. Oh how wonderful that He answered my prayers. He delivered me from my fear and doubt and from being sorry for myself, to being blessed that I am in His Hands. My body is His temple! He lives in me! He alone gives and takes life. He alone knows the life span for every human being. No one else! I have to live my life to the fullest, as I do battle to win over my cancer. I have strong faith in Him. My whole being is secure in His love. I will face my tomorrow with courage, peace and confidence. I look forward to the many exciting opportunities that He will open for me to express my unique personality as His child. My life is in the best of Hands. Praise the Lord!

"Find rest, O my soul,

in God alone;

my hope comes from him."

(Psalm 62:5)

Joyful
Hope

I had my first chemotherapy on March 10, 2005, four weeks after surgery. Although my doctor discussed with me the possible side effects of the anti-cancer drug, I was overwhelmed at how my body reacted. After four hours of chemotherapy, I felt worn out. I was sleeping in the car as my daughter drove us home. Upon arriving home, I went straight to bed. It seemed I had no energy. I felt very tired. That night, I experienced shooting pains all over my body especially in my stomach area. I had a burning sensation all over my body, especially on the soles of my feet. My muscles ached and my neck was stiff and painful. My scalp was tender and my heart beat faster. Four days later, my lips began to crack and I had small skin blisters that looked like acne on my face, chest, neck and head. I had quite a lot of difficulty hearing a person's voice over the phone. I had constipation, which aggravated my hemorrhoid. My vagina was dry and painful. My taste buds were not functioning.

I felt very tired each day, and every night I prayed to God to help me endure the pain and to give me the strength to carry on. I was determined to regain my strength, therefore, I made sure that I got enough rest, ate balanced meals and nutritious snacks, had daily devotions and exercise. I also took some medicines prescribed by my doctor to alleviate some of my pain.

The side effects began to gradually diminish after ten days; however, on the fourteenth day while taking my shower, lots of hair came out and fell on my face, neck, shoulders, over my body and onto my feet. When I felt the hair on my fingers, I cried out loud! I continued crying as I tried to wash the hair off my face and other parts of my body. My loud cry competed with the noise of water coming out from the showers. My tears mingled with my hair as I was trying to wash them off. I prayed loudly to God. "Lord, I knew this would happen but I did not expect that it would be so soon! I know this is just hair and it will grow back but it still hurts to lose it. Please help me to accept this and all of the other side effects. I want to get well. Help me to endure my pain. Please give me the strength to live one day at a time. I praise You for whatever You will do for me."

It seemed like an eternity when I was finally able to wash off all the hair from my body. I felt clean and refreshed. As I stepped out of the bathtub, I felt like God's Hands were helping me step onto new ground, a ground that was solid and secure. I also felt like I was a new person, one who had joyful hope and quiet resolve to work toward my complete healing and wholeness.

"Look to the Lord

and

his strength;

seek his face

always."

(Psalm 105:4)

Fear

and Serenity

My chemotherapy treatment schedule was every first week of the month. Before my first treatment, I asked a lot of questions of my doctor, regarding the side effects of the anti-cancer drug. He answered all of them with confidence. Since I had not undergone any treatment I was a little bit scared and anxious and at the same time curious as to how my body would react to the drug. I went to my first chemotherapy with a positive attitude. It was after my first experience that I realized how much pain I had to endure for days due to the side effects. I experienced over-all bodily fatigue, muscle pain, tingling and burning sensations, sore neck, constipation, sores in my mouth and blisters on my body especially in my chest area. Through prayers and strong determination to get better, I weathered each day until the painful side effects seemed to have diminished and I began to feel better.

As my second chemotherapy treatment was approaching which was April 6, 2005, my fear and anxiety level began to rise. I was just beginning to feel better and soon I would be undergoing another treatment. I dreaded those painful side effects on my body all over again. I wanted to delay the schedule of treatment but I knew this was unrealistic. I had to go through it as scheduled. These feelings of fear and anxiety caused me to lose sleep.

In order to help me further understand myself, I called my friend who had colon cancer. "I felt anxious and fearful, too, each time I had chemo," she said. "I even cried," she added. "My husband told me to look at it this way; the earlier I complete my treatment, the closer I am to my healing." She shared that she and her husband prayed to God everyday and asked Him to give her strength and comfort. "I will be praying for you that you will be strengthened and comforted by our Lord," she concluded. I thanked her for her encouragement and for praying for me.

By the grace of God, a friend from Los Angeles whom I have not heard from in years called after she found out about me from a relative. "I am calling you to let you know that ever since I received the news, I have been praying for you. Trust in the Lord, my dear friend." She told me that she had breast cancer and had a mastectomy. She admitted her fear, anxiety and other negative thoughts and knew too that these would not help her in her healing. She said that through constant prayers her negative thoughts and feelings dissipated slowly. She also shared that by thinking of the fun times she had with her husband and young daughter and the future fun times that they would have together helped her to accept her pain with positive feelings. "God carried me through. I am now cancer free," she announced happily. I thanked her for strengthening my faith and for her surprise call, which meant so much to me.

My friend from New York also called because a mutual friend wrote to her about me. To my surprise, she told me that several years ago she also had a hysterectomy but it was not cancerous; however, a year ago she found out she had breast cancer and underwent a mastectomy. She had been taking pills called tamoxifen and will do so for the next five years. She also underwent breast reconstruction surgery. "I thank Jesus daily that I am alive. I am thankful that God has extended my life and I continue to enjoy my family," she said. "Do not fear, but be thankful," she advised me. We promised to continue praying for one another.

My friends' testimonies definitely lifted my spirit. They took Jesus' words with them during their painful moments and during their recovery. They focused on God! And how about me? I failed to focus on Him all the time. I focused more on the impending pain that I would be experiencing, rather than on God's comforting words. The thought of pain engulfed my serene spirit. I failed to look up to God who had assured me when I began my journey toward recovery that He would never leave me. God had not left me. It was I who had left Him! I realized that even though I am His child I could easily forget His promise of deliverance if I was not focused on Him every second of every minute. I was vulnerable like everyone else. I felt like I experienced what Saint Peter, one of Jesus' disciples, experienced when he failed to fix his eyes on

Jesus. He wanted to walk on water like Jesus. He was able to do it as long as he fixed his eyes on Jesus, but when he began to focus on his surrounding, he began to sink. (Matthew 14:25–30) This was true of me, too. I lost sight of God and focused on myself. I also lost sight of the things that my friends shared with me about their constant awareness of God's presence during their ordeal. I prayed humbly, "Dear Jesus, please forgive me for my failure to focus on You all the time. I have to look up to You moment by moment and nothing else." After praying I breathed a big sigh of relief, with a grateful heart. I knew that my friends' testimonies and specially their prayers helped restore my serenity.

"Dear friends,

since God so loved us,

we also ought to love one another.

No one has ever seen God; but if we love one another,

God lives in us

and

his love is made complete in us."

(1 John 4:11–12)

Connected

through God's Love

It was about 5:30 in the afternoon when I heard the front door open. It was my son who had just come home from work. "Mommy, you have some mail again. It seems you get some mail everyday," he said happily as he handed it to me. I eagerly took it and went to sit down in the living room. It always made me happy to receive something in the mail.

My face brightened when I opened the first one. It was a combined graduation and birthday announcement from a former student who attended our school in Kindergarten along with her two siblings. She would be graduating from High School. Her beautiful invitation included three pictures of herself, when she was a baby, a little girl and a graduating senior. "What a beautiful girl she has become! I would certainly not be able to recognize her if our paths would cross someday," I said to myself. The invitation included a dinner party at one of the fanciest hotels in Waikiki. I was very happy at her accomplishments and thankful for her inviting me on this special occasion.

The second was a wedding invitation from another former student who attended our school when she was also in Kindergarten. She wrote a personal note in the invitation telling me that she and her future husband were looking forward to meeting me. The wedding reception would be held at one of the best hotels in Waikiki. I was deeply touched that she remembered me through these many years and wanted me to meet her future husband.

The third was a package from a friend whom I met several years ago when I was a volunteer helping foreign students at the East-West Center. She lives in New Jersey with her family. "Here is a journal for you. Fill up the pages with your poems. Thank you for all that you have done for me. I will be praying for your quick recovery," she wrote. I was glad that God had directed her steps through the years.

The fourth was from a former participant of the support group for the divorced, widowed and separated, which I had facilitated for several years. She wrote to say that I was in her thoughts and prayers. She also said, "I thank God for all the ways He has used you in the lives of countless people, and your ministry of helping the broken-hearted. My friend, I do not know why God has given you this cross to bear but I know that He walks with you and loves you with His everlasting love. You will always be in my prayers." I was pleased to note in her letter that her faith in Jesus remained strong in spite of her emotional pain and brokenness.

The fifth was from a colleague. "There are many people praying for you. You have touched many lives and we love you. God knows your needs and He will be with you and give you comfort, peace and assurance. Our faithful Lord will walk with you as your health is restored. I will keep praying for you." I was happy that she loves her work and continues to serve God.

The sixth was from my niece. She happily shared, "We attended Benny Hinn's Miracle Healing Crusade in Manila. We claimed healing and fast recovery for you. Long life and good health to you. Glory to God who loves you very much. We will continue to pray for you. We love you always." I was grateful that she continues to love God with gladness.

Surely their loving thoughts, good wishes and prayers are affirmations of their love which brought joy to my heart. I tried to recall some events that made me enjoy their unique personalities. There were vivid memories of a talented five-year old girl being nurtured by her loving and hard-working parents along with two other children; a bright and beautiful young pre-teen who was learning how to cope and develop friendship relationships with her peers; a courageous young lady who wanted to take some calculated risks to follow her dreams; a newly divorced young woman who was very determined to do all she could to meet the needs of her young children and herself; a hardworking colleague who loved her work helping students and their parents; and a family member who has been delighted in sharing God's love since she was a young girl.

I said a short prayer for my blessings. "Lord, thank You for these special people in my life. Their warm thoughts and prayers for me, especially during this time of my life, give me great joy. I love them, so please continue to bless them as You also bless me."

It is during my recuperation that I came to fully realize the many connections I have with so many people because of the love we have for one another. It amazes me to see the many expressions of love through cards, post cards, letters, gifts, pictures, e-mail, phone calls, etc. Technology has certainly made it even easier for relatives and friends from foreign countries, across the United States and in Hawaii to send wonderful messages of love, hope, encouragement, and prayers.

My daughter, who lives in Los Angeles, calls or e-mails me almost everyday asking how I am. "I love you, Mommy. Do not worry about me because I am trying to arrange my schedule so I can come and see you soon!" she said in her last e-mail.

My mother-in-law, who lives in Massachusetts, called and said, "I wish I could be there with you for a few days. I think of you everyday and I will be sending you something that will bring me closer to you, knowing you will read the same words that I have read and getting the same help I have. I love you and take care of yourself." A few days later, I received a booklet of inspirational poems that helped strengthen my resolve to get better.

Family members here and abroad kept asking how they could help further. Their prayers and support remained strong. It was the same with my friends.

"My whole family is praying for you! Let us know how we can help," e-mailed a friend from New York.

"We are saddened to hear about your illness, but God is in control. He will see you through. We will keep on praying for your full recovery. We regret that we can not be there to visit you but we will continue to pray daily," said a couple from Texas that I dearly love.

"We always pray for you during Sunday school. We look forward to seeing you back in church," said my Sunday School teacher.

I also found out that other churches in Hawaii had included me on their prayer lists. I was also being prayed for by friends during their mid-week Bible Study and Intercessory Prayer meetings. One of the pastors wrote and said, "Greetings in the powerful name of our Lord Jesus Christ. Tonight at our prayer time, we lifted you up to our Lord in a special way. Remember, God who knows our trials and sufferings is always there for us. He is the Great Physician and He knows your every need and He will bring healing to your body and soul."

Indeed I felt so much loved by so many people. Each one of them means so much to me and I thank God for all of them. The love, support, prayers, and kind deeds that several of them had shown me in the past helped me to become who I am today, a committed child of God.

As I thought of love, I came to think of the doctors, nurses, aides and other caregivers who lovingly helped me get back on my feet at the hospital. Oh how I admired their patience and words of encouragement during my painful ordeal. They had smiles on their faces as they attended to my needs. They are like angels on earth. I shall always be grateful for their excellent caring of patients and unselfish devotion to duty. I will always be connected to them.

Through my life's journey I have come to a full realization that my major goal in life is to love God, and if I love Him, I should keep on loving people no matter how imperfect I am. I am still growing in this area; however, I know that God will help me as I share His love with others. He wants me to show kindness, compassion, goodness, thankfulness, cheerfulness, forgiveness, honesty, joy, peace and hope to others. Of course I had negative experiences with some people, too, because of anger, fear, hate, unforgiving attitude, jealousy and impatience; however, through God's grace and mercy, I have come to accept and work on my inadequacies and have asked forgiveness from people I have hurt and offended. I have also asked God to forgive me whenever I stumbled in following His footsteps. I have asked Him to continually show me how to grow in His love, because my ardent desire is to continue obeying Him. Everyday I have asked Him to help me see myself through His eyes. I know deep in my heart that every step I took that brought me closer to Him has been a wonderful experience. Many times I have also asked Him to help me become more sensitive to people and to continue learning how to overcome my weaknesses and value and use my strengths. While I continue to grow in loving Him, I have come to realize that every experience, whether negative or positive, has helped define who I am as a person and as a child of God. My spiritual connection with Him has tremendously helped deepen my relationship with others in my role as a mother, sister, ex-wife, daughter-in-law, aunt, principal, co-worker, friend, and volunteer.

It grieves me that several special people in my life have passed away. These are my beloved parents, brother, and some friends; however, their love and positive influence in my life will always be in my heart. Their love makes me connected with them forever!

My connection with people through God's love is also true with people I do not even know. This realization became so evident when my son and I went to Ala Moana Beach Park one Sunday afternoon. I felt love toward those families having picnics under their tents, the young and old people who were playing frisbees, biking, swimming, surfing, jogging, reading, sleeping, etc. I love them with brotherly love because they are created by God just as I am. And as I looked toward the ocean as far as my eyes could see, I visualized the many people in the other parts of the globe whom I felt connected with, because they are also created by God. I am part of humanity just like they are. I also came to recall my friendship relationships with former classmates from different countries like the Philippines, Japan, Thailand, Indonesia, Cambodia, Nepal, India, Sri Lanka, Mongolia, Australia, Malaysia, South Korea, Ghana, Scotland and the United Kingdom. I felt connected with them because they had shown me love and I love them. I will always cherish the happy memories I had with them.

Although I am connected with so many people there is one connection that is stronger and more lasting, my connection with family members, friends and other people who are also my brothers and sisters in Christ. This strong bond is due to the fact that we have the same unforgettable life changing experience of receiving the Holy Spirit in our hearts when we accepted Jesus Christ as our Lord and Savior. Our connection is beyond family relationship and friendship, because we are connected spiritually through the Holy Spirit. Our love for the same God binds us together not only on earth but also when we will come to the end of our life's journey and will be with our Lord in heaven forever.

I remember when I received six letters from a church in Oklahoma, the First Baptist Church of Moore. I was excited to find out who sent me those letters because I did not know any one from this church. As I read them, I found out that they came from Christian people who had heard from one of my Christian friends about my ordeal; therefore, they wrote to send me their love and encouragement. One of them said, "I have not heard your name before but my heart goes out to you and my prayers go to our loving Father. I am sure you have read 'Footprints in the Sand'. This will be the time when He will be carrying you through your ordeal. There will only be one set of footprints. You have been a good and faithful servant. We pray that your health will be restored." She signed, "Your sister in Christ, Willie." I felt connected with her and her friends because we love, worship and serve the same Lord. Although we have not met personally, she loves me as her sister in Christ and wants the best for me. We are bonded by God's love because we are God's children. We belong to the family of God.

I have many family members and friends whom I respect and love dearly but they do not know the Lord. I long to be connected with them on a spiritual level because it would make our relationship even more special. We could share how the Holy Spirit is leading us in our everyday lives. I will continue to pray for them that one day they may come to know God's saving power and, therefore, experience the joy of a transformed life, a life that is peaceful and joyful through Jesus Christ. I pray that I would be one of those people who would lead them to Jesus Christ.

I feel so blessed to be surrounded by people who love me. I feel I have a similar experience as the Israelites when they were in the wilderness on their way to the Promised Land. They had no food and they prayed to God who showed His great love and mercy by giving them manna from heaven everyday. This manna nourished them and they did not die. (Deuteronomy 8:15–16) Similarly, I am also in my wilderness experience because of my cancer and I pray to God to help me in my journey toward complete healing. I know that my family and friends are praying for me, too. Our prayers are like manna from heaven that continue to strengthen my faith, comfort my soul, and sustain my hope and positive attitude for a bright future. I praise and glorify God each day for the many special people with whom I am connected through His love.

"Pray without ceasing."

(1 Thessalonians 5:17, KJV)

Peaceful Heart

My room at the hospital looked like a florist shop. It was filled with beautiful floral arrangements sent by friends, students and their parents, co-workers, and colleagues. The sweet fragrance that enveloped the room helped me to focus less on my pain due to surgery. As I read the cards, I visualized the faces of the senders and the special moments I had with them. I felt happy that they were praying for me and were sending their love and good wishes for my early recovery.

During my recuperation, I received cards, letters, drawings, books, pictures, CD's, video tapes, cooked meals, food baskets, floral arrangements, and other gifts. I was overwhelmed by the continued expressions of love, concern and support for my children and me.

Every night I prayed. "Lord, thank You for my family, friends, my school, my church, and my support group. Thank You for the comfort and strength that You give me each day. Please help me to get better and help my children and me as we go through this journey of healing together."

In order to help me have a productive day as much as possible, I made up a daily schedule. It included a time for the following: Bible Study, meditation, reading, writing, watching Christian shows and news on TV, watching funny shows on DVD's or videos, exercise, and short naps. Everyday I looked forward to following my schedule but I seldom finished everything that I listed because I did not have enough energy and I took longer naps.

One of the things that gave me excitement was reading and looking at the letters, cards and drawings of the students, which were over 500 in all, excluding the cards and letters from family, friends and colleagues. Everyday, I would take a few and read them.

"Mom, you have so many people who love you. You are a cherished woman!" my daughter commented as she was reading some of the students' letters. We both admired many of the students' drawings and pinned some of them on my bulletin board in my bedroom. I treasured all the items I received and filed them neatly inside my drawer. Each one was like a tiny pearl given to me for safekeeping.

The many messages of love warmed my heart.

"All of us miss you at school. Come back soon so you can see our happy faces!" wrote a fourth grade student.

"Get well soon so we can hear your stories during chapel," wrote a fifth grade student.

"We miss you teaching us math. I like Math. Please return soon," wrote a first grade student.

"We raised $218.33 for the tsunami victims by selling food and toys. I am sure that if you were here, you would also help us. We will continue to pray for you and the tsunami victims," wrote another fourth grade student.

"Did you like my drawing? I drew it just for you," asked a first grade student. She drew a huge pink heart surrounded by tiny pink stars with bold pink words written across, "Get well soon!" She drew herself and me facing each other smiling surrounded by small light blue flowers.

"Thank you for helping my children. You are more than a principal to my family. You are our mentor," wrote one parent.

"You're sorely missed by my class. We will wait patiently for your return. God loves you and so do we," wrote one teacher.

"We made you a special DVD about our students. We hope that this brings a smile to your face. We missed you participating as usual in the children's activities. The children and I continuously pray for you. Jesus loves you," wrote another teacher.

"We missed you visiting our class. The children and I look forward to your coming back. We pray for you each day. Here are some pictures of the children during our Field Day," wrote another teacher.

"My mom has the same sickness as you do and she asked God to heal her. God will do the same for you. My mom and I pray for you daily. I can hardly wait for you to come back so I can give you a big hug," wrote a third grade student.

I felt blessed each day as I continued reading these letters and cards from people who are special to me. Then one day, when my children went off to work, I felt sad! I missed my work, too! I missed dressing up nicely and driving my new car to go to work. I missed seeing the happy faces of the children and watching them playing happily on the playground. I missed helping and teaching them. I missed working with the teachers and other administrators. I missed conferencing with parents and helping them with their concerns. I missed eating lunch with the children and teachers at the cafeteria. I missed attending chapel and watching the children sing and participate actively. I missed leading the Bible devotion with the secretaries during the week. Oh, how I missed being at school and being a part of an active and loving community that reaches out to our parents and students. I missed doing the job that I loved so much for over thirty years! I yearned to be with them. I felt that I deserted the children and the people I love working with. I felt very sad! "Lord, please do not let me feel sad," I prayed. "Help me to live one day at a time so that I can bear this feeling of sadness of not being useful." I never thought that I would have this feeling of sadness. I tried to look at my situation objectively but somehow this feeling persisted. I know that God is in control of my situation and I have to trust in Him because He knows what is best for me.

I tried to overcome my sadness by watching funny videos and reading some books. It helped a little. At night when I said my prayers, it seemed God was far away and I could not reach Him. "Lord, I do not want to be cooped up at home. I want to be where the action is, at school. How can I serve You in my condition?" I cried quietly as I lay in bed feeling despondent.

My son noticed my lack of pep. "Why are you not eating? You hardly touched your food. Come on, eat so that you will get stronger," he said and he added more food in my plate. I told him how difficult it was for me, a very active person, to be suddenly cooped up a home. I told him how I missed my work. Upon knowing this, he said, "God wants you to focus on yourself at this time so you can help your school later. You are no good to parents and students and even to your teachers if you are not well. Nobody wants a sick principal. I am sure your school will understand. It is not that you are being selfish to think of yourself first; it is just being realistic. So get busy by keeping yourself fit!"

What he said was true yet I could not erase the feeling of sadness that kept lurking in my heart. "Lord, please settle my heart and mind. This feeling is robbing me of joy," I prayed silently as I forced myself to complete my exercise routine.

Then one afternoon, something happened that changed me. I came across these letters from students at our middle school.

"You helped me a lot. You prayed for me when I was in the hospital in first grade. Now is my turn to pray for you. I hope you become better because one of your greatest joys is to help students," wrote a seventh grade student.

"Thank you for praying for me when I was in second grade. I was going through a hard phase concerning my family then. You came to my classroom and held my hands and we prayed. Every time I saw you after that, you gave me a hug and asked how my family and I were doing. It was really comforting to know that someone cared about my feelings and thoughts. I appreciate all the prayers and good wishes you have sent out for me and my family. I still think of you and the wonderful things you have done for me. I hope you get through right now, whatever you have. I will be praying for you," wrote an eighth grade student.

"Thank you for praying for me and for not kicking me out of school because of the trouble I caused you. You gave me grace. I have changed now. I've matured and have become hungry for knowledge. My lowest grade is B-. There is one person I should thank and that is you. I will be one of many who will be praying for you. I know you will get better because God is still using you to help other kids that were like me before. You have already changed hundreds of lives including mine. Thank you for changing my life," wrote another eighth grade student.

After reading these, tears welled up my eyes. I felt so blessed that the prayers I had with them when they were little made a difference in their lives. How would I have known then? Now, they are sharing it with me. These beautiful souls are growing up in the Lord. How wonderful to be used by God. What a blessing!

Suddenly I realized that I stopped praying for others since I had the surgery and now that I am recuperating. How did I miss this very special will of God for me to pray unceasingly? I have to continue praying for those children I had been praying for, even before my surgery. Under no circumstances should I stop this special will of God for His children. I prayed silently. "Thank You, Lord, for bringing me back to Your fold. Thank You for revealing to me through the letters of these children that I can serve You by praying unceasingly for others. My responsibility is to pray and You will handle the rest."

As I continued reading more and more letters and cards, my whole being felt light. My lonely heart became a peaceful heart!

"I will praise you, O Lord,

with all my heart;

I will tell of all your wonders.

I will be glad and rejoice in you;

I will sing praise to your name,

O Most High."

(Psalm 9:1–2)

Song
of Praise

On June 14, 2005, at 7:00 p.m., I was back in the emergency room at Kaiser Hospital in Moanalua. Only four and a half months ago, I was admitted here complaining of intense pain on the left side of my abdomen and two days later I underwent surgery, total hysterectomy with the verdict of ovarian cancer. This time, I was complaining of intense pain on the right side of my abdomen, especially when I breathed in deeply! My son and I were very anxious to find out what was causing this sudden pain. We thought I was recuperating very nicely from my first surgery and also doing very well with my chemotherapy; therefore, this change of events was highly unexpected.

After all the tests were completed, Drs. Payne, Weber and Abcardian came to talk with my son and me. They informed us that I had an infected gallbladder and the operation would be done once I got stronger. In the meantime, Dr. Abcardian will put a stent in my gallbladder to drain some pus so as to lessen my pain. As I was being prepared for this procedure, my son and I held hands. I could see his troubled countenance, so I tried to smile to calm him down, and said, "Do not worry. I will be fine. God is in control." He followed the nurse and me to the cat scan room. Once there, he sadly bade me goodbye. A few minutes later, Dr. Abcardian performed the procedure, while I was still in the cat scan machine. He used the cat scan images to guide him. At the beginning of the procedure, I felt a dull pain in my abdomen; however, as I began to drift out of consciousness, I prayed silently, "Lord, please have mercy on me! Please guide this doctor's hands. Please be with my son and me. Thank You that we know now what was causing my pain."

When I woke up from the procedure done by Dr. Abcardian around noon time, I found that I was in a small room by myself. I saw IV's on both my hands. I called for a nurse and asked what the IV's were for. She told me that I was being fed intravenously, since I would not be given food without the doctor's orders. The other IV's were medicines to alleviate my pain and to take away my infection and fever. She instructed me how to press the small button when I wanted more relief from pain.

When she left, I felt so saddened and weakened at what was happening to me. Here I was, lying in a hospital bed connected to IV's and being prepared for yet another surgery! I felt overwhelmed. I cried! I felt so alone. I prayed to God earnestly. "My dear Lord, please take care of me. I trust in You, Lord."

His affirmation to my prayer came instantly and in the most simple and beautiful way. Outside my bedroom, through the glass window, I saw two small brown birds hopping around the branches of a big tree, looking for food. They seemed content and even having fun at what they were doing. I watched them for a long time and soon I began to feel calm. Suddenly I realized that these birds are God's creation and He takes care of them. (Psalm 136:25) He will certainly do the same for me!

The following day, Dr. Chan, the oncologist who was in charge of my chemotherapy, came to see me and shared that my blood pressure and white cell counts were low. He assured me that he would do all he could to help me, but one of the things that must be done was for me to have a blood transfusion. He assured me of the safety of this procedure; therefore, I gave my consent. He also told me that my chemotherapy treatment would be postponed, because of what I was going through. Before he left, I thanked him for his caring attitude.

Soon after Dr. Chan had left, the hospital minister, J.P., came to visit me. He also visited and prayed for me twice when I had my first surgery. It was comforting to see him again. He gave me a book of Psalms and then led the prayer. "Our precious God and Great Physician, I humbly ask that You watch over Mrs. Ovitt. Please comfort her now and be with her when she will have her surgery. Please strengthen her body specially at this time. Please give her that special peace that only comes from You. May you also comfort her children who love her very much. Please be with her doctors and others who are helping her. We pray for these things in the mighty name of Jesus, Amen." Before he left, I thanked him for visiting and praying for me again.

That afternoon, two male nurses came to give me my blood transfusion. They made sure that the numbers on the plastic pouch containing the blood were the same numbers written on my wristband. They called out the numbers three times. Once assured, they went ahead and completed the connection of the IV to me. When they left, I watched intently and silently as the blood was flowing through the white plastic tube into my vein. I kept watching silently. As I did this, my thoughts went to those 'loving people' who donated their blood for others, including me. Before I knew it, tears wet my face. I prayed to God to bless these kind donors and thanked 'them' from the bottom of my heart for donating their precious blood to save my life. I am blessed by their unselfish giving. As I continued looking at the blood flowing steadily into my vein, I also began to think of God's blood that washed away my sins. Jesus shed His blood on the cross at Calvary for me, so that I would be saved and have eternal life. (Ephesians 1:7)) I am blessed forever.

My surgery was scheduled for 8:30 in the morning of June 17, 2005. My daughter flew in from Los Angeles and made it on time to be by my bedside before I was taken into the operating room. She prayed for me, "Dear Jesus, please be with my mom. Please be with the doctors, also. My brother and I love her very much. Please give us assurance that everything will be alright." Before she left, she squeezed my hands, kissed me on the cheeks, gave me the sweetest smile and assured me that she would be waiting outside until the operation was finished. I was ready for the surgery. Once again, I put my life in God's loving Hands.

When I woke up that afternoon, I felt an excruciating pain in my chest and abdominal area. I had a big gauze that covered my seven-inch incision, beginning about three inches below my right breast and slanted toward my right abdomen. I had two small plastic tubes inserted in my nostrils that provided me more oxygen. There was also a small pouch that was catching some blood that was coming through a small hole from my right side. I had a catheter inserted and was wearing leg massagers. When my daughter came to check up on me, she saw that my left arm was swollen, due to the many blood samples having been taken. Immediately they took out the IV's and put a midline catheter in my right arm to help alleviate my pain. My door remained closed, to give me peace and quiet. I slept most of the time, because I felt very weak and tired. Phone calls were blocked and visitors were not allowed, except for my children and those they approved of. In the midst of my pain, I repeatedly prayed in my mind, "Our Father" (Matthew 6:9–13) and "The Shepherd's Prayer" (Psalm 23:1–6) until I fell asleep.

When Dr. Payne came to see me he had a big smile on his face. "The surgery went well and no cancer! We took out your very infected gallbladder with this many stones," he said as he cupped his hand. "Now you can begin to heal." His good news lifted my spirits. He continued telling me that at first they did a laparoscopy, the most common procedure that uses small incisions; however, when they saw that my gallbladder was so infected, they did open surgery. In this procedure, they made an incision in the abdominal area to remove my gallbladder. When the doctor left, I shook his hand and thanked him and the other doctors for the fine job they had done to make me better. Although there was still severe pain, my heart was singing praises to God for the good news.

I shared my joy with my children and ex-husband when they visited me. They were equally joyful. My ex-husband led the 'thanksgiving prayer' to God before they left. "Our most gracious and heavenly Father, we thank You for this wonderful news that there was no cancer in the gallbladder. We thank You for the successful surgery. We thank You for her doctors and nurses. Please comfort her and give her strength so that she will get stronger each day and can return home soon. Help us to continue to support her in her healing." When I went to sleep, my heart was at peace.

As each day passed by, I kept counting my blessings, especially the loving and caring people around me. And one special blessing is my small room with a fantastic view! God is so kind to let me see a tiny slice of His creation. He knew just how to soothe my aching body. Through the glass window, I could see big, healthy, beautiful trees. Some of them had large white flowers while others were covered with vines that have bright, clustered yellow flowers. I could see birds and butterflies flying around. At a distance, I could see this huge pink medical building, the Tripler Army Medical Center, and the cars that passed by in front of it. And most of all, I could see the gorgeous deep blue sky with its huge foamy clouds. As I looked at the beautiful clouds, my imagination took over. I came up with some creative images such as a gondola, the dome of St. Peter's Basilica, the spire of the cathedral of Milan, the top of the Leaning Tower of Pisa, a part of the Roman coliseum, a statue of an angel, a cross, a lion, lake, hill, mountain, etc. These were some of the places that my daughter and I visited in Italy. As I created more images, time seemed endless. I was lost in the moment of my creation. I experienced such wonderful freedom of expression that I forgot my bodily pain. I was thoroughly one with nature. What an awesome feeling!

While I was still in my imaginative-creative mood, my thoughts brought me to the fact that life is fleeting, just like those images I had created. They vanished in a split second with the slightest movements of the clouds. Life is precious. Life is a gift. Each moment is a treasure to behold. I have to live my life fully, even when I am sick. Life is now. I have to make my life count for God in whatever circumstance I am in.

Suddenly, I came to think of the Apostle Paul, who preached boldly about the saving power of Jesus Christ, even though his life was threatened wherever he went. He never lost sight of his single mission in life, that of sharing God's salvation for everyone. He was a passionate witness, wherever he went, even when he was in prison. His strong faith in God is a great testimony for all believers! (Ephesians 3: 7–8) Just like him, I have to share God's wonderful love and grace right where I am, in my room. I immediately prayed to Jesus, "Lord, please make me a blessing to others. My illness should not keep me from sharing about You. Help me not to waver in my expectation that You will use a broken vessel like me. Help me and teach me to grow in You."

An opportunity came the following morning when a new lady came to take my blood pressure. She was accompanied by her supervisor, who was watching her intently as she performed her task. She was very nervous during the whole process. In the afternoon, she came back to take my blood pressure again. "Hi! I am glad to see you," I said. I sensed her nervousness as she began to do her work. I told her to wrap the blood pressure cuff tighter, because it was quite loose. She apologized as she unwrapped it. It was much better the second time. She told me that she was nervous because it was her first day of work! "I will pray for you," I told her and patted her shoulder. "God will help you become better each day." She replied softly, "Thank you very much!" When she left, she waved and smiled at me from the door. When she came to take my blood pressure the following day, she told me right away that she prayed to God to help her, even before she started her morning duty. I praised her for doing so and assured her that God helps those who help themselves. From then on, each time she came to take my blood pressure, she was more confident and we also had a small friendly chat. After taking my blood pressure in the morning on the day I was discharged, she quietly took my hand and said, "Thank you for your encouragement and prayers. I am not nervous anymore. I like my work because I meet different kinds of people." I thanked her for helping me and commended her for being dedicated in what she was doing. I will always remember the way she waved and smiled at me from the door.

I was amazed at how each day's experience brought me closer to Him. Everyday this lady helped me to have my dry bath. She would lovingly and carefully get me out of bed then gently lead me to the bathroom where she would help me have my dry bath using special disposable wash cloths. She would help me dry my body with a towel and put on a new gown. Once done, she would help me sit down on a chair next to my bed. She would then kneel down, wash my feet, dry them and put on new socks. Each day that she did this, I wanted to cry. I felt so touched deep inside. I have never done what she was doing to me to someone else except to my children when they were little. What she did reminded me of the Last Supper when Jesus washed the feet of His disciples. He wanted to give them an example that they should also wash one another's feet. (John 13:4–5; 12–17)

I always thanked her profusely after each bath. She would just smile and say, "I am glad you feel better." As I lay down in bed I prayed, "Oh God how You remind me of Your loving kindness through this beautiful lady. How refreshing to experience love from someone who gives of herself freely for others. I know it is part of her job to help me but she gives it so lovingly. May You give me opportunities in my remaining life to serve You with a compassionate and humble heart just like her."

One day I noticed her sadness and I asked why. "My mother is sick but she still has to baby sit. I can not get another babysitter and even if I do, I can not afford to pay. I will have to be absent from work if she continues to be sick." I told her that I fully understood her problem because I faced it, too, when my children were little. "Why don't we pray right now and ask God to heal your Mom and provide a solution," I suggested. She readily agreed. The next day, she told me that her husband took off from work to take care of their baby and the following day was her turn. I was surprised to see her back. With a big grin and hands clasped to her chest she exclaimed, "God is good. Our prayers are answered. My mother is better and is babysitting." Her face glowed as she was exalting Him. It looked so beautiful. On the last day she was helping me, I was surprised when she asked me to pray for her beloved mother who is 72 years old. She shared how deeply she loved and appreciated the big help that she gives to her and her family. I promised her that I would. We hugged as we bade goodbye. I will never forget the lesson God taught me through her.

When Dr. Cynthia Weber, a young and beautiful resident intern at Kaiser and Tripler Army Medical Center came to visit me, she praised me. "You look like a million dollars! If I were to compare you with my male patient who is much younger and had the same surgery as yours, I can say that you are much stronger and healing faster." I replied, "Thank you for your encouragement. I ask God to heal me and give me strength everyday and He does. " She did not make any comment about what I said. As we talked I found out that she was from South Carolina and would be graduating from the University of Chicago's medical school in 2007.

On the day I was discharged, she came to check me one last time and to remove the small pouch that hold some blood that was draining from my right side. She said, "Good luck and keep up with your breathing exercise." I promised her that I would. I also told her that everyday whenever I looked at Tripler Army Medical Center from my room that I always offered a prayer to the Lord for her, to guide and direct her steps as a resident intern and to achieve her goal to become a surgeon. I also told her that I thought she would become an excellent surgeon. She did not say anything when I said these things but she gave me the sweetest smile. When I saw her smile, I immediately added, "Please smile more often. You are a beautiful doctor and when you smile your patients will feel more relaxed. Also, you have such a nice set of teeth. Don't be too serious. I hope I will see you someday. God bless you and keep you." When she left the room, she said with a smile, "Keep exercising and keep that positive attitude!" In my heart I knew that I was blessed by her dedication to her profession. I will continue to pray that she will be used by God, the Great Physician, as she helps her present and future patients.

I was required to do my walking exercise everyday and my daughter was always delighted to help me. We would walk to the nurses' information desk then return to my room. This one afternoon though, we walked all the way to the lanai and admired the natural beauties surrounding the hospital. On our way back, we found a small chapel with beautiful stained glass windows with the image of Jesus Christ. We went in and sat down. We were absorbed by the quietness around us. Then my daughter reached for my hand, bowed and prayed. "Dear Jesus, please make my mom stronger each day. Please heal her wounds from her two surgeries. Please heal her cancer, too. My brother and I love her very much. We need her." In silence, we continued holding hands. I felt God's presence and my heart was overflowing with joy. A little while later, she got the Bible and read aloud Psalms 23 and 91 while I bowed my head and listened. What she read reminded us that God is our refuge and fortress and we will fear no evil because He is with us all the time. When we left God's pretty little house, I felt so close to my loving God and to my daughter.

I was discharged on June 22, 2005, at 1:00 o'clock in the afternoon. My daughter and I were delighted that I was going home. As she was getting final instructions from the nurse outside, a social worker came into my room and asked if there was anything else I needed. I told him that I wanted more information about my surgery for my file. He went out and came back with the literature. As he was about to hand me the papers, he saw me putting my Study Bible in my bag. He asked, "Are you a Christian?" I replied proudly, "Yes, I am." He immediately replied, "Me too!" We both smiled at each other as we shook hands. He shared openly that he came to know the Lord after his painful divorce. It was God who carried him through his crisis. God has blessed him with a good job, a Christian wife and a good church. As he talked, I could see peace in his face. He then looked at the pages of my Study Bible and was surprised to know that I continued studying in spite of my surgery. I told him that I had to continue to learn God's words so that I could share it with others. I also told him that I asked God to use me while I was in the hospital. Then he said, "I wish I could do the same. I need to discipline myself daily to study His Words. I also want to share Him with others. " I answered right back, "He will help you with your heart's desire. Your obedience and willingness will be honored by Him. He will do the rest. Why don't we pray right now?" He replied readily, "Yes, let's do it." We held hands, bowed our heads and prayed. "Our Father, thank You that my brother and I can pray together right now. We are Your servants, Lord, and we praise You and honor You for being our loving God. Lord, at this time, I ask that You continue to bless my brother. Please help him in his desire to learn more about You and also to share You with others. May Your Holy Spirit empower him so that he can bring joy to many people's hearts. In Your precious name we pray, Amen." Before he left, he gave me a big hug and said, "I am glad I have met you and we prayed. I will be praying for your speedy recovery." When he left, I quickly gave thanks to God for allowing me to meet him. I felt blessed.

As my daughter pushed my wheelchair toward the elevator, I was praising God for all the wonderful experiences I had had during the past few days. He had lifted my spirit, touched my soul, nourished my body, and used me to share His love. Nine days earlier when I came I was reaching out to Him for mercy and now that I was leaving, I was holding a cup of blessings. And my cup is overflowing!

"In everything give thanks:
for this is the will of God in Christ Jesus
concerning you."

(1 Thessalonians 5:18, KJV)

Thankful Heart

One of the beautiful things in Hawaii is the weather. The temperature is usually between 70–85 degrees Fahrenheit. Everyday when I woke up at around 8:00 o'clock a.m., I would open the front door to let the fresh air come in to fill the apartment. The fresh air helps in my healing. Then I would go and stand by the south lanai and enjoy the beautiful blue skies, the beautiful garden with well trimmed trees of the next door condominium and the verdant mountains at a distance dotted with a few big beautiful homes. After feasting on this view, I would go and stand by the north lanai and enjoy some view of the Waikiki skyline and the Pacific Ocean, and again the vast blue skies with its foamy clouds that cover the island of Oahu. I continue to be awed by the beauty of God's handiwork. I am blessed and thankful to God that I live in Honolulu, one of the most beautiful cities in the United States.

One afternoon at around 4:00 o' clock, I decided to go to Makiki District Park instead of doing my breathing exercises at home. It has been seven months since I had my two surgeries, a hysterectomy and the removal of my gallbladder, and I have not visited this park recently. I missed this place that holds a special place in my heart. I excitedly put on my walking shoes, shorts, soft white jacket, and a nice blue cap to cover my bald head. I had walked to this park a hundred times before and it usually took me about fifteen minutes to reach it, but this time, it was taking me so long. The soles of my feet were numb, one of the side effects of the cancer drug; therefore, I could not walk fast. I had to make sure that my steps were steady otherwise I might stumble. I also had to rest midway because I was tired.

Upon reaching the park, familiar scenes and places greeted me; such as the happy children playing on the playground, energetic young men playing kickball on the front lawn, some families sitting on mats talking and taking naps under the beautiful trees, several gardeners tending to their plants at the community garden, joyful children and adults swimming in the pool, teams of young people fiercely competing at the basketball and tennis courts, and book lovers at the library.

I felt good to see the many active people, because their energy seemed to rub off on me. I also felt good to remember the happy times my children had at the playground when they were little, the many friendship relationships that we had developed in this place through the years, and the hard work that we put into caring for the plants in our little plot at the community garden, as well as our excitement and happiness whenever we harvested vegetables like lettuce, green onions, beets, tomatoes, beans, and eggplants for family and friends. This place is a haven of happy memories.

As I continued walking, I felt energized when my feet touched the thick, dark green grass. I began to walk faster and enjoyed the bouncy, happy feeling. It was the same feeling that I had when I stepped out of the car and walked toward my apartment after being discharged from the hospital for each surgery. I was back at home! I was thankful to God for helping me overcome my surgeries and facing my recovery with calmness.

When I walked by the plumeria trees I smelled the sweet scent of their beautiful blossoms, which were white with a tint of yellow at the middle. There were hundreds of wilted and fresh blossoms on the ground. I picked some fresh blossoms, smelled them and put them gently inside my pockets. As I did this, I came to think of the sweet love of Jesus as He held me tenderly close to His heart when the doctor told me about my cancer of the ovary, when I had to go for chemotherapy treatments, when I had my infected gallbladder taken out, and when I had my divorce.

I remember when I sought my Pastor's counsel during one of the lowest points in my life, my divorce. He told me, "Our God is omniscient. He has infinite knowledge and He knows what you are going through. He loves you very much and I know you love Him, too. Put your full trust in Him. He has a very good plan for you. In everything give thanks." (1 Thessalonians 5:18) I asked him why I should be thankful when my heart was bleeding and breaking because of intense emotional pain. He explained, "It is God's will for us to be thankful in every circumstance in our life. He is not asking us to be thankful for our tragedies. He does not want you to be thankful for your divorce, but He wants you to be thankful for what He could provide you in your heart-breaking circumstance. You could thank Him for His love, compassion and guidance in the midst of your pain. He is in control of all circumstances, including yours. He will also give you peace and joy in your suffering, if you remain close to Him."

I was illuminated when I left his office. God wanted me to thank Him in everything, not for the crisis I had, but for what He had provided me in my painful experience. I immediately gave Him thanks for His faithfulness. I felt my aching soul was lifted up!

Now I am facing the most crucial circumstance in my life, my battle to conquer ovarian cancer. I do not thank Him for my battle but I thank Him for giving me strength, courage, joy and peace in facing it. I have strong faith in Him. He is holding my hands as I combat this disease boldly and confidently. I continue to pray that He will bestow upon me His loving kindness throughout our journey together.

As I smelled the blossoms in my hands, He gave me His sweet affirmation to my prayer as He whispered softly to my heart, "I am with you. Nothing can separate us because I love you and you love me." I gave Him a hearty "Thank you!"

"Be still,

and know that I am God;

I will be exalted among the nations,

I will be exalted in the earth."

(Psalm 46:10)

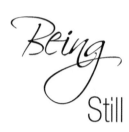

Being Still

I could hardly wait for these dates to come, September 6, 2005, when I would have my blood test and a meeting with Dr.Chan, my oncologist; and September 7, 2005, when I would have my last chemotherapy treatment, according to the schedule.

Before these dates, I received e-mails, phone calls, letters and cards from family and friends in Hawaii, other states, and abroad, expressing their continued support, encouragement, and prayer, as I reached the last cycle of my chemotherapy treatment. Just like me, they were delighted that my chemotherapy treatment would soon be over. I eagerly looked forward to resuming the job that I love, being an elementary school principal, and continuing to conduct a support group with the Bible Institute of Hawaii for the divorced, widowed and separated. I had been recuperating at home for eight months due to my two surgeries and chemotherapy treatments and I missed my school, church, and the many wonderful people who had been supporting and praying for me.

"The whole school is praying for you during flag everyday. We miss you and we will keep on praying for your recovery", said our vice principal when we talked over the phone.

"Every night I pray for you. I hope you will get better and I will see you soon. I love you. Thank you for teaching me Math in first grade. I hope you like my picture", said a second grader in her letter along with her beautiful drawing of her and me together.

"Hopefully soon we will be able to hug each other on Sunday mornings. You are truly missed", wrote a dear friend from church.

"Thinking about you all the time. My prayers are for you that the Lord gives you strength and peace. It's a hard long journey but remember we are with you and God never fails", wrote a dear friend who is also battling cancer.

"We are rejoicing in the Lord that your chemotherapy treatment will soon be over. We pray for you everyday. Keep your faith and never stop praying to Jesus. He loves you very much and we do, too", said my loving sister who called from the Philippines.

"I can hardly wait to help you again when you will start a new support group. Our friends and I continue to pray for you and look forward to being with you", said a dear friend who has helped me for several years.

"I have prayed for you everyday, at Sunday mass and my visits to the Blessed Sacrament at our Perpetual Adoration Chapel. I have also called our church in Pearl City because I wanted to offer a mass for you on Sunday", said a long time friend.

The lovely thoughts and committed prayers of special people in my life lifted my spirit. I felt calm. I was physically, emotionally, mentally, and spiritually ready for my last chemotherapy treatment.

My check-up with Dr. Chan on September 6, 2005, went well. He informed me that my blood count was good; therefore, I would proceed with the chemotherapy treatment. He told me that I would be given Taxotere, just like in my fifth treatment, instead of Taxol, because I still had numbness in the soles of my feet and in the palms of my hands. He also told me that after my last treatment, he would be seeing me every three months for the next five years, to find out if the cancer cells would return. Both of us hoped that they would not and I would be healed completely. Furthermore, he said that I would be able to resume my work on December 5, 2005. Praise the Lord!

I shared what Dr. Chan told me with Dwight, my ex-husband, when he came to pick me up. He was delighted that my journey toward healing was going well. It was God's grace and true forgiveness that were keys to our emotional healing and becoming friends. He had been helpful to the children and me, especially during my illness.

That night I was excited as I prepared all the things I needed. I took the list that I had used previously and put check marks on the things I had done or made ready for the following morning. The list included the following: lunch, snack, fork, napkins, water bottle, paper, pen, eye glasses, devotional, iPod, visa card, Kaiser card, walking shoes, warm socks, wig, long pants and the matching top, hat, jacket, earrings, necklace, ring and watch. This time, I added a camera because I wanted to take some pictures on this special day.

After I had finished my Bible study and evening prayer, I went to bed. I closed my eyes and thought of that night before my first chemotherapy treatment on March 10, 2005. I was very anxious and a little scared then, because of the unknown, but tonight my feeling was different. I was excited, happy and thankful that my last treatment was about to happen and although I knew the side effects that I would have to endure, I was not scared. My whole being felt light and my mind was at peace.

While lying quietly I could hear my own breathing; the faint noise of the wind passing through the slightly opened glass louvers of the front door; and the gentle rustle of the leaves of the tall trees in the neighbor's yard as the wind caressed them. I kept lying still and in those precious peaceful moments I could feel His Holy Presence. I could feel His warmth and I felt so blessed. I felt so loved. I closed my eyes and prayed, "Lord, how marvelous is Your love for me. Thank You for sustaining me through my surgeries and chemotherapy treatments. I know that my journey toward complete healing has its own time. It is according to Your time, not mine. Thank You for my family, friends, and many others who love and support me. Please bless them as You bless me."

The following morning, September 7, 2005, I was ready by 7:00 o'clock. I had my shower, a light breakfast and all the things I needed in one beautiful bag. My son dropped me off at Kaiser Hospital, Moanalua, at 8:00 o'clock on his way to work. As we bade goodbye, he gave me a big hug and said, "I love you, Mommy. Be brave and do not think of the side effects." I smiled at him then walked toward the Oncology Clinic.

As I entered the new and beautiful Chemotherapy Treatment Room, I was greeted with big warm hugs by Mrs. Debbie Casuga and Mrs. Diane Nakagaki, who helped me in my previous treatments and were also former parents of my school. They knew it was my last treatment and they were happy to see me doing so well. I had some pictures taken with them and immediately after, they started the treatment procedure for me. As the long needle went into a vein on the back of my left hand, I closed my eyes and offered a silent prayer, "Oh Lord, please put Your loving arms around all of us here so that we can taste Your wonderful peace and grace and delight in Your comfort and strength."

About thirty minutes later, the lady on my right side turned on the TV to watch the news. It was about the catastrophe brought by Hurricane

Katrina to the states of Louisiana and Mississippi. "Oh how horrible! Look at that devastation!" she exclaimed. I looked and saw the unforgettable images of the floodwater covering the once livable land, the uninhabitable homes, the hundreds of homeless people and the very busy and tired rescue workers. "Those poor people are fighting for their lives! And we are fighting for ours, too! All of us need hope!" she said emphatically. I looked at her and said, "I agree with you." She looked at me and smiled and I smiled back. Soon we were sharing about ourselves.

How true what she said! Hope, gently and lovingly wrapped in prayers, is needed by the homeless, displaced, broken-hearted, disadvantaged, at-risk and afflicted people. It is the beacon of light for the hopeless. It propels them to be creative and use their inner strength to overcome their bleak situation, because a bright future was waiting on the horizon. And in this treatment room, it is hope that binds all of us together. We were all afflicted with one disease, cancer; and hope, along with prayers, will give us the strong resolve to overcome our affliction and to become healthy again.

As part of this group, I could feel the survivor's instinct in all of us. I could say without a doubt that no one among us wanted to be losers, but be winners. We were not cowards, but brave souls fighting for our lives. We were taking our treatments in our own quiet and dignified way and with courage and determination. Although we were seated about three feet away from each other, we were aware of each others' pain and shared in each others' feeling of relief, when one of the medicinal pouches in our respective IV stands was removed and was replaced with a new one. It meant nearing the end of treatment! We shared quiet happiness when someone had finished her treatment. When these words, "thank you" and "goodbye" were said before she left, we experienced joyful anticipation that soon it will be our turn to say these special words, too. The one who had finished her treatment was somehow viewed as a conqueror; she had conquered the enemy, the cancer cells, courageously! However, soon after we had heard those parting words, we also began to accept the reality that another courageous person was seated on the recently vacated comfortable couch, and thus the process of treatment repeated itself. Perhaps this made us all the more awake to the realization that Life had to go on, whether inside or outside of this room. We had to meet its challenges in whatever circumstance we were in, with our heads up, calm spirits and God's leading.

As the hands of the clock continued to move on, the room became even quieter because several of us were either sleeping or resting, due to the side effects of the cancer drug. I continued to be awake and listened to

Christian and Hawaiian music from my I-Pod and read my devotional book. However, about three hours into my treatment, I became tired and sleepy, too. I wanted very much to continue what I was doing, but my body began to slowly succumb to the drug. I came to think of the story of the disciples, Peter, James, and John when they were with Jesus in the Garden of Gethsemane. Jesus asked them to keep watch while He went to pray, but they were not able to stay awake, although they were willing. They were tired and fell asleep. (Matthew 26:36–41) I could identify with how those disciples behaved, because there were times when the body just needs rest.

At around 1:30, a dear friend came to pick me up. I tried to be awake on the way home. She offered a prayer before she left me. I thanked her for praying and appreciated her loving kindness and helpfulness. I went to bed immediately and when I woke up, it was about 8:00 o'clock in the evening. My son forced me to eat and drink a lot of water. I tried with the little energy I had.

In the next few days, I faced the challenge of overcoming the side effects of the cancer drug with quiet endurance. I tried to be positive. I was resolute in taking some positive actions that would improve my physical strength, maintain my emotional stability, nurture my peaceful and happy thoughts and keep my heart burning with love and thankfulness for my compassionate and gracious God.

After two weeks, my bodily pain had gently and greatly diminished; therefore, I decided to walk around my neighborhood. I used to do this before but now that my chemotherapy treatments were over, I wanted to make it a daily routine. I wanted to get better and stronger so that the cancer cells would not come back.

Before my illness, starting from my apartment, it usually took me about thirty minutes to walk around six blocks by three blocks. I wondered how much time it would take me now. I marked September 21, 2005, with a big red star on my calendar as the beginning of my regular walking exercise. At around 5:00 o'clock that afternoon, I headed toward the elevator and as I pushed the button for the first floor, I prayed silently for God to give me strength and to keep me safe.

I felt happy when I passed by the familiar homes, apartments, condominiums, schools and churches and saw the different kinds of trees, shrubs, vines and other varieties of plants in their gardens, yards, hedges and fences. I was delighted to see these different fruits again: banana, pomelo, coconut, noni, tangerine, papaya, mango, guava, passion fruit, avocado, etc.

I enjoyed seeing these beautiful flowers again: the flaming red, orange and yellow hibiscus; the white, red, orange, dark and light purple bougainvillas; the white and purple vanda orchids; the yellow bird-of-paradise; the pink and red torch ginger; the yellow heleconias; the white tube rose; the small red and white anthuriums; the white gardenia, etc. And of course, I had to stop to smell my favorite flower, the dainty, white and sweet pikake blossoms growing by a fence. How refreshing to see all of these beautiful living things. I missed them. I love my neighborhood.

I came to think of the thousands of neighborhoods that were wiped from the face of this earth due to natural disasters, like earthquakes, tsunamis and hurricanes. I have continued to pray for the displaced people in Asia, Louisiana, Mississippi, Florida and Texas. I could not even imagine their intense pain and suffering because of their losses. As I walked, I prayed, "Oh Lord, please surround those broken-hearted people with Your love, comfort, and strength. Please guide them as they make crucial decisions because of the enormous challenges that they are facing everyday. May they continue to look up to You because You are in control of the whole situation. May their hope remain high and their faith strong as they try to put their lives back together. Please help and bless also the many people who are reaching out to them." I could surely identify with them. We were all broken-hearted and we needed healing from the Lord.

When I reached the end of the sixth block, I felt exhausted! I sat on the edge of a planter's box facing the very busy Punahou Street. I tried to catch my breath. I felt pain in my legs. I realized that I had over exerted myself. I should have planned for a shorter walk. I massaged my legs and stamped my feet.

While I was massaging my legs and stamping my feet, it occurred to me that I did these too when I joined the Holy Land Tour with 84 pilgrims for two weeks in March 1993! Several of us massaged our legs and stamped our feet each time we rested after our long walks to see some historical and holy places such as: Mount of Olives, Palm Sunday Road, Garden of Gethsemane, Church of the Nativity in Bethlehem where Jesus was born, House of Caiphas, Tomb of King David, Temple Museum, Upper Room, Wailing Wall, Masada, Dead Sea, Qumran, Pool of Bethesda, Via Dolorosa (Way of the Cross), the Church of the Holy Sepulcher which now stands over Golgotha, Garden Tomb, Valley of the Shadows, Jericho, Nazareth, Cana, Magdala, Jordan River, Capernaum, Mount of Beatitudes, Sea of Galilee, Megiddo, Mount Carmel and Caesarea. We felt pain in our legs and feet but we did not complain because of the awesome and unforgettable experiences we had. We walked where Jesus walked! Several of us cried when we were re-baptized at the Jordan river and after each short and moving worship service in the places where Jesus was born, had His Last Supper, carried the cross, was crucified, buried and resurrected! Our Bible teacher and leader ended his last sermon by asking us the same question that Jesus asked Peter, "Do you love me?" (John 21:17) My answer then and even now was, "Yes, I love You. You are enthroned in my heart forever." I long to return to this very special place with my daughter someday and I hope that God will give me another chance.

One very special and vivid memory happened when we walked in the Old City, Jerusalem. The streets were narrow and very crowded! Someone could easily get lost there. Our tour guide told us that if we were lost, it was better to return to the hotel rather than look for the group. He told us that it had happened several times that someone was lost; therefore, we should always look at the red flag that he was holding up high so that we would be able to follow him and not get lost.

As I was being pushed by people around me trying to follow our tour guide, I suddenly remembered the story about Jesus and His disciples when they were walking in this same place. A woman who had been bleeding for twelve years touched Jesus' cloak from behind and her bleeding stopped instantly. Jesus asked His disciples who touched His clothes. He knew it was a different kind of touch. His disciples told Him that because of the crowd, they could not tell who had done it. When He looked around, the fearful woman admitted what she had done. Jesus told her that because of her faith she was healed. (Mark 5:25–34)

This woman's story of faith and healing, even though it happened many years ago, had become "alive" and had touched me deeply. Both of us loved Jesus Christ. Both of us wanted healing from our affliction. Jesus healed her and I sincerely believe that what He did for her then, He would do for me. My Jesus is alive and His Words have power and remain forever.

I had the urge to pray and although surrounded by noise from the vehicles passing by, I stilled myself and bowed my head, "Oh my Jesus, I want my healing, too, just like that woman who touched You and whom You healed many years ago. My faith is in You, dear Jesus, and I believe in Your miracle of healing. Thank You for hearing my prayer." After praying, I had peace in my heart.

The much needed rest energized me. I continued walking and I recognized a neighbor who just got off the bus. There was also a neighbor who waved at me while driving and I waved back. Both of them were coming home from work.

My cancer and where I am in the stage of my life had changed my perspective about work. For several years I worked very hard to achieve and perform well in my job and to provide material things for my family. I was given recognition for my hard work and dedication. Somehow slowly, there was a change taking place in me; achievement and having worldly possessions were no longer top priority. Now, I wanted to focus more on myself. My "doing" was now secondary to my "being"; focusing on what else I could discover about myself. I wanted to fully realize myself. I wanted to become that unique person God wants me to be. This process of becoming is a beautiful adventure with Him.

As I came closer to my home, I saw several people whom I had met before such as the lady who colors the long white fur of her dog, Rosie, pink; the elderly lady who always greets me with a big smile; our former maintenance man who is always cheerful; the couple who walk holding hands; the nurse who walks with her patient; the lady who had heart surgery; the grandmother who walks with a cane; the hardworking mother who drives a limousine; the teacher's aide who works in the nearby school; the beautiful college student; and the smiling Math teacher. I waved at some of them and they waved back. It was a great feeling to see them again.

It was getting dark so I walked briskly and then I saw the tall, beautiful shower trees with their thick green leaves and countless long hanging clustered blossoms and past them was my apartment building. What a lovely sight, their pinkish-yellowish loose petals strewn over the sidewalk and street and a stream of petals steadily and slowly falling down to the waiting earth. The soft wind played with them and they twirled and danced as they fell down.

As I walked underneath, some loose petals gently touched my head and shoulders. I felt marvelous! Suddenly I came to think of the blessings that God poured out on me when I was in the emergency, operating, recovery and chemotherapy treatment rooms! Oh how He gave me strength, comfort, courage and assurance that He would be with me all the way. He wiped my tears and took away my fears and anxieties. The constancy of His love made me still. Although I was physically weak, I felt strong inside; although suffering I could rejoice. Only a few months ago, I was lying in the hospital suffering and now I was about to finish my first walk in my neighborhood! It was all because of His amazing mercy and grace. Tears welled up in my eyes and soon

I was crying because of thankfulness. I felt so grateful and rich because of His abundant blessings!

When I arrived at the entrance of my apartment, I stilled myself and wiped my tears. As I opened the gate with my key, I also opened my heart to God and asked Him to please continue to work out His plan in me. I look forward to many exciting adventures with Him because my joy is in serving Him. My life is in Him and I will go forth with gladness and courage because I know that He lights my path. I am secure in His faithfulness and abiding love. How wonderful to be a child of God!

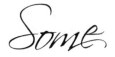

Bible Verses That Were Helpful to Me

When I was angry:
Psalm 4:4 "In your anger do not sin; when you are on your beds, search your hearts and be silent."

When I was anxious:
1Peter 5:7 "Cast all your anxiety on him because he cares for you."

When I needed assurance:
Psalm 23:4 "Even though I walk through the valley of the shadow of death, I will fear no evil, for you are with me; your rod and your staff, they comfort me."

When I needed courage:
Deuteronomy 31:6 "Be strong and courageous. Do not be afraid or terrified because of them, for the Lord your God goes with you; he will never leave you nor forsake you."

When I cried:
Psalm 61:1–2 "Hear my cry, O God; listen to my prayer. From the ends of the earth I call to you, I call as my heart grows faint; lead me to the rock that is higher than I."

When I was depressed:

Psalm 34:18 "The Lord is close to the brokenhearted and saves those who are crushed in spirit."

When I was discouraged:

Deuteronomy 31:8 "The Lord himself goes before you and will be with you; he will never leave you nor forsake you. Do not be afraid; do not be discouraged."

When I had doubt:

Jeremiah 32:27, KJV "Behold, I am the Lord, the God of all flesh: is there anything too hard for me?"

When I wanted assurance of eternal life:

John 3:16 "For God so loved the world that he gave his one and only Son, that whoever believes in him shall not perish but have eternal life."

When I wanted God's love and faithfulness:

Psalm 108:3–5 "I will praise you, O Lord, among the nations; I will sing of you among the peoples. For great is your love, higher than the heavens; your faithfulness reaches to the skies. Be exalted O God, above the heavens, and let your glory be over all the earth."

When I had fear:

Isaiah 41:10 "So do not fear, for I am with you; do not be dismayed, for I am your God. I will strengthen you and help you; I will uphold you with my righteous right hand."

When I needed forgiveness:

1 John 1:9 "If we confess our sins, he is faithful and just and will forgive us our sins and purify us from all unrighteousness."

When I wanted healing:

Isaiah 53:5 "But he was pierced for our transgressions, he was crushed for our iniquities; the punishment that brought us peace was upon him, and by his wounds we are healed."

When I felt helpless:
Psalm 5:1–3 "Give ear to my words, O Lord, consider my sighing. Listen to my cry for help, my King and my God, for to you I pray. In the morning, O Lord, you hear my voice; in the morning I lay my requests before you and wait in expectation."

When I felt hopeless:
Isaiah 40:31 " . . . but those who hope in the Lord will renew their strength. They will soar on wings like eagles; they will run and not grow weary, they will walk and not be faint."

When I was lonely:
Psalm 42:5 "Why are you downcast, O my soul? Why so disturbed within me? Put your hope in God, for I will yet praise him, my Savior and my God."

When I needed love:
John 15:9 "As the Father has loved me, so have I loved you. Now remain in my love."

When I needed mercy:
Psalm 116:1–2 "I love the Lord for he heard my voice; he heard my cry for mercy. Because he turned his ear to me, I will call on him as long as I live."

When I felt needy:
Philippians 4:19 "And my God will meet all your needs according to his glorious riches in Christ Jesus."

When I wanted peace:
Philippians 4:7 "And the peace of God, which transcends all understanding, will guard your hearts and your minds in Christ Jesus."

When I thought of God's plan for me:
Jeremiah 29:11 "For I know the plans I have for you, declares the Lord, plans to prosper you and not to harm you, plans to give you hope and a future."

When I wanted to praise God:

Psalm 9:1–2 "I will praise you, O Lord, with all my heart; I will tell of all your wonders. I will be glad and rejoice in you; I will sing praise to your name, O Most High."

When I wanted to quiet my heart:

Psalm 46:10 "Be still, and know that I am God; I will be exalted among the nations, I will be exalted in the earth."

When I thought of my relationships with family, friends and others:

Romans 12:9–13 "Love must be sincere. Hate what is evil; cling to what is good. Be devoted to one another in brotherly love. Honor one another above yourselves. Never be lacking in zeal, but keep your spiritual fervor, serving the Lord. Be joyful in hope, patient in affliction, and faithful in prayer. Share with God's people who are in need. Practice hospitality."

When I thought of my salvation:

Psalm 62:1–2 "My soul finds rest in God alone; my salvation comes from him. He is my rock and my salvation; he is my fortress, I will never be shaken."

When I needed strength:

Psalm 46:1–2 "God is our refuge and strength, an ever-present help in trouble. Therefore we will not fear, though the earth give way and the mountains fall into the heart of the sea, though its waters roar and foam and the mountains quake with their surging."

When I thought of thankfulness:

Ephesians 5:19–20 "Speak to one another with psalms, hymns and spiritual songs. Sing and make music in your heart to the Lord, always giving thanks to God the Father for everything, in the name of our Lord Jesus Christ."

When I needed to trust:

Proverbs 3:5–6 "Trust in the Lord with all your heart and lean not on your own understanding; in all your ways acknowledge him, and he will make your paths straight."

When I felt weak:

2 Corinthians 12:9–10 "But he said to me, 'My grace is sufficient for you, for my power is made perfect in weakness.' Therefore I will boast all the more gladly about my weaknesses, so that Christ's power may rest on me. That is why, for Christ's sake, I delight in weaknesses, in insults, in hardships, in persecutions, in difficulties. For when I am weak, then I am strong."

When I felt weary:

Matthew 11:28–30 "Come to me, all you who are weary and burdened, and I will give you rest. Take my yoke upon you and learn from me, for I am gentle and humble in heart, and you will find rest for your souls. For my yoke is easy and my burden is light."

How

Does One Become a Christian?

I would like to share with you how one can become a Christian, how I became a Christian and others, too. This may help you understand and decide to become one.

To become a Christian, you have to:

1. Accept that you are a sinner.
2. Confess your sins to God and ask for His forgiveness.
3. Believe that Jesus Christ is Lord and He died for your sins on the cross. He saved you from your sins.
4. Ask Jesus to come into your heart and tell Him that He is Lord of your life.

When you do these, God's Holy Spirit will come and dwell in your heart. It is then that you have become a Christian, a child of the living God! As a Christian, your Lord and Savior is Jesus Christ, no one else. You are now assured of an eternal life in heaven with Jesus.

These are the Bible verses that support how one becomes a Christian.

John 3:16 "For God so loved the world that he gave his one and only Son, that whoever believes in him shall not perish but have eternal life."

Romans 3:23 "For all have sinned, and fall short of the glory of God."

Romans 10:9 "That if you confess with your mouth, 'Jesus is Lord' and believe in your heart that God raised Him from the dead, you will be saved."

Romans 10:13 "For everyone who calls on the name of the Lord will be saved."

When I was fifteen years old, we were studying in Sunday School Matthew 6:33, KJV "But seek ye first the kingdom of God, and His righteousness; and all these things shall be added unto you." I asked my teacher what "these things" mean and she said that these are things that are good for me, things that are not harmful for me and others. My teacher further added that if I wanted "these things" I have to seek God's kingdom but most important of all, I have to become His child first. I have to accept that I am a sinner, confess all my sins to Him, and then ask Him to come into my heart. I should also believe that Jesus Christ loved me so much He died for my sins so that I would be saved.

As a fifteen-year-old, I wanted God to help me to have good friends and become a good student therefore, when our pastor asked who wanted to become a Christian during the time of "Invitation", I went forward and knelt in front of the altar. I talked to God quietly and said, "Dear Jesus, I am a sinner and I confess all my sins to You. Please forgive me. I believe that You died for my sins on the cross and I thank You for saving me. I want You to be my God from now on. Please come into my heart, Lord Jesus." After saying this, I felt joyful and I had tears of happiness. His Holy Spirit came and lived in me at that moment. I became a Christian! Jesus became my Lord! God answered my prayers and many more through the years; I have continued to serve and glorify Him.

Please note that you can become a Christian at any age, time and place, with or without someone helping you.

A friend shared with me how he became a Christian. He said that he accepted Christ as his Lord and Savior at the beach at 5:00 o'clock in the morning. He said that he raised his hands toward the sky and shouted: "Lord, I believe in You. You died for me. I am a sinner. Please forgive me of all my sins. From this day onward, I want You to be my Lord and Savior." He said that after doing this, he felt tremendous peace and he knew that the Holy Spirit had come into his heart. He is now very active in his church.

A few years ago, I shared with a friend who attended my support group for the divorced, widowed and separated how to become a Christian, inside my car in a parking lot. After knowing how, she said that she wanted to accept Jesus as her Lord and Savior right then! We held hands and bowed our heads. She spoke, "Lord, Jesus Christ, I want a peaceful life. Please take over my life from now on. I have sinned against You and others so please forgive me of all the sins that I have committed. I want You to be my God from now on. I want to love You and obey You." We were both crying after this. She told me later that after she became a Christian, she became a much happier and peaceful person. She also found her life more meaningful.

God is waiting for you to become His child. If you are not yet a Christian, I pray that you will accept Him as your Lord and Savior now.

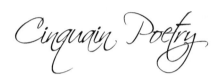

Alopecia

ugly, dreadful

crying, objecting, questioning

I felt very sad.

Hair loss

Birthday

happy, memorable

singing, dancing, hugging

Wishing 'wishes' come true.

Natal day

Cancer

malignant, virulent

penetrating, devastating, unsettling

I'm fighting it courageously.

Disease

Insomnia

restless, sleepless

turning, walking, imagining

I felt very tired.

Wakeful

Operation

risky, scary

debilitating, enervating, encapsulating

I let go of fear.

Surgery

Prayer

devotional, intercessional

praising, petitioning, communicating

I feel so peaceful.

Worship

Shower

helpful, delightful

refreshing, caressing, rejuvenating

My strength is returning.

Quick bath

Telephone

quiet, useful

ringing, singing, clamoring

Time to make connection.

Phone

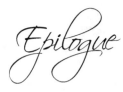

A Cancer Patient's Prayer

i

Lord, how can I forget that memorable day

When my doctor said to me gently,

"You have ovarian cancer, the aggressive type."

I sat quietly.

Then I felt Your warm hands touching mine.

I heard You whisper softly,

> "I am here. It is alright. I will not leave you!"

I accepted my physical condition silently and completely.

Suddenly I felt

> Your peace,

> Your strength and

> Your comfort.

I felt secure.

ii

My dear Jesus, as I go through my journey of healing,

Please stay close to me.

     I want to feel Your warmth.

Please hold me.

     I want to feel Your empowerment.

Please bathe me with Your radiant light.

     I want to feel Your serene spirit.

I pray to You earnestly to restore my body.

Please hear the prayers of

     your humble servant.

     your faithful disciple.

     your loving child.

iii

Lord, please help me when sometimes these intense feelings come:

     fear and anxiety of pain and the unknown,

     anger at not being in control,

     loneliness of being isolated, and

     discouragement for being inactive.

These feelings

     consumed my quiet thoughts;

     enveloped my peaceful soul;

     disturbed my calm spirit; and

     sapped my renewed energy.

Lord, please

      forgive me for dwelling in these incapacitating emotions and

      deliver me from them.

      bestow upon me Your grace and mercy.

      wipe my tears with Your tender hands and

      cleanse me with Your forgiveness.

Lord,

      I praise You.

      I thank You and

      I love You!

iv

Oh God, I am surrounded by love.

Thank You for my

      family,

      school family,

      church family,

      support group,

      friends,

      colleagues,

      doctors, nurses, and other people that I do not even know

      You sent my way

      to help me.

Thank You Lord for their

      love,

      prayers,

support,

kindness,

compassion and

encouragement.

Thank You that I am loved. I feel

loved,

content,

joyful and

blessed.

Their love comes from You

For You are LOVE!

V

Oh Lord, You know me intimately.

You know my

blessings and disappointments,

successes and failures,

dreams and longings,

gifts and losses,

strengths and weaknesses,

hopes and fears,

joys and sorrows,

challenges and temptations,

goals and obsessions,

accomplishments and short comings, and

brokenness and new beginnings.

You know my

> past,

> present, and

> future!

You have control of my life. I belong to You.

I trust You! I have faith in You!

> You know me.

> You created me.

> You love me.

vi

Lord, thank You that

> I am saved by Your grace.

> I have everlasting life.

> You love me forever.

I have surrendered my

> body,

> soul, and

> spirit

> to You!

I sing praises to You! You are my

> Comforter,

> Redeemer, and

> Everlasting Father!

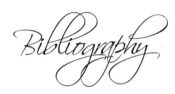

Bibliography

General Editor, Baker, Kenneth; Associate Editors, Burdick, Donald; Stek, John; Wessel, Walter; and Youngblood, Ronald. **The NIV Study Bible New International Version.** Grand Rapids, Michigan: Zondervan Bible Publishers, 1985.

The Holy Bible
Cambridge, At the University Press
Great Britain

Edited by Gardner Associates. **Who's Who in the Bible.** Pleasantville, New York Montreal: The Reader's Digest Association, Inc., 1994.

U.S. Department of Health and Human Services, Public Service, National Institutes of Health, National Cancer Institute, **Chemotherapy and You (A Guide to Self-Help During Cancer Treatment),** September, 2003.

CPSIA information can be obtained
at www.ICGtesting.com
Printed in the USA
JSHW011719040919
1228JS00003BA/6